Mediterranean Diet for Beginners

Everything You Need to Get Started. Easy and Healthy Mediterranean Diet Recipes for Weight Loss

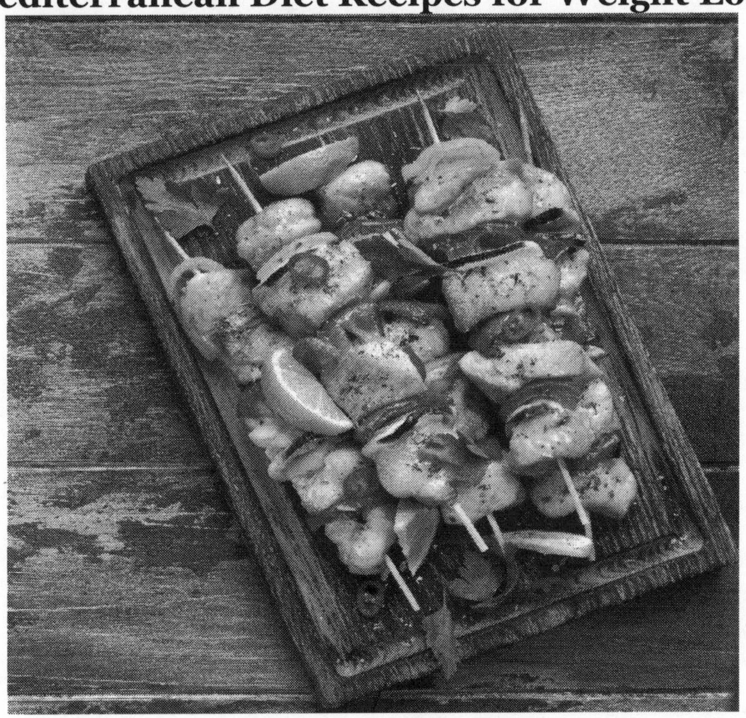

Brandon Hearn© 2019

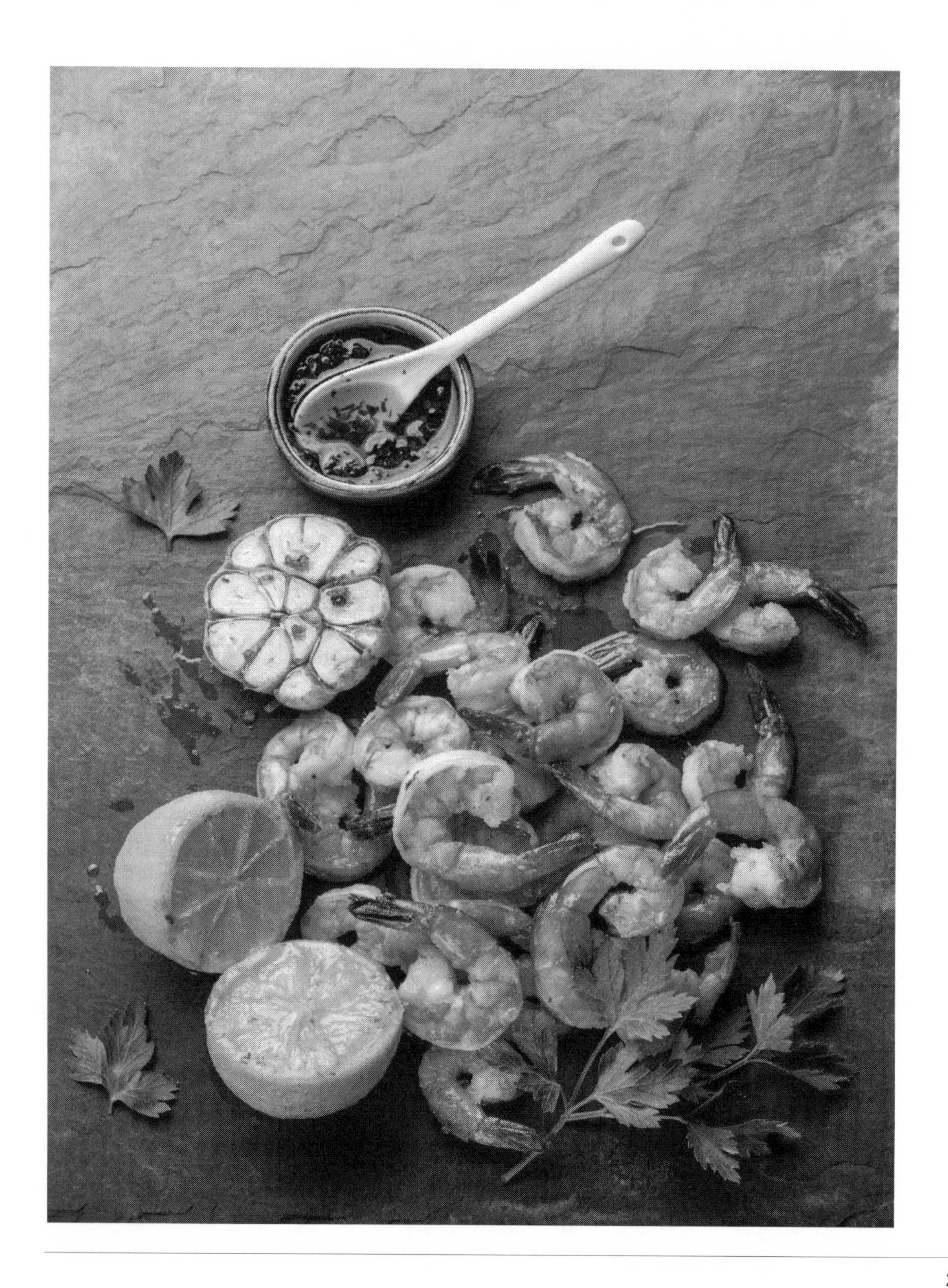

Table of Contents

Introduction

Before you can start your health and weight loss journey with the Mediterranean diet, you need to understand what it really is. To do that, let's take a brief look at the history and science behind the diet to explain why it really works. The ingredients in this diet will help you to meet your health goals as well as your weight loss goals. You'll also learn the many benefits that the Mediterranean diet has to offer.

The History Behind It

This is a nutritional model that's been formed through studying the dietary patterns of a typical Crete person. Of course, the diet has evolved through the years, but it's closely related to the Mediterranean lifestyle as well as the culture, territorial, social, historical, and environmental aspects of those people. It isn't new, and that's where the strength in this diet lies.

It's early origins even incorporated the Biblical seven species which were barley, grapes, figs, wheat, pomegranates, date honey and olives.

These foods as well as other foods of the Middle East are now recognized scientifically as health foods that can help with your heart health as well! However, the typical person doesn't live like a Crete.

Currently we have an increased calorie intake along with decreased physical activity which ahs put our health in jeopardy which leads to disease and obesity sky rocketing.

Fat intake has also increased while there has been a decrease in fiber intake. As a people we now consume more complex carbs and less vegetables and fruit. Cardiovascular disease and cancer have been three times higher than in the Crete people. Meals are often eaten in front of the TV, which encourages overeating and 1quick meals, which means we have to adopt healthier habits.

The Health Benefits

Now, we can discover some of benefits that the Mediterranean diet has to offer!

- **Reduced Risk of Cardiovascular Disease:** There is a correlation between cardiovascular disease and diet from different parts of the world. Ancel Keys discovered a clear relationship between a decreased level of cholesterol and the prevalence of coronary heart disease due to the Mediterranean diet. This is because the Mediterranean diet includes many vegetables, fresh fruits, olive oil, garlic, red onions, herbs and other foods that have a vegetable origin. There is only a moderate consumption of red meat too. The fresh and natural ingredients of the Mediterranean diet is that they have more minerals and vitamins than the processed food that has become so common.
- **Longer Lifespan:** Those living on the Mediterranean coast have the longest lifespan, and it isn't a coincidence. The climate ensures and abundance of vegetables, fruits, beans, fish and olives which are high in antioxidants. Antioxidants combat aging which can be triggered by pollution and stress, which is high in the Western world. Antioxidants also help to fight against inflammation which can lead to chronic disease such as cancer and heart disease. The bit of DNA located at the tip of chromosomes is referred to a telomeres, and they shorten every time a cell divides. They can

shrink by half from infancy to adulthood, and then they shrink again by half for the elderly. However, those that eat a Mediterranean diet have been known to have longer telomeres.

- **Weight Loss Help:** The Mediterranean diet alone may not be enough for instant weight loss, but it will certainly help you along the way. When paired with physical activity and portion control, it can help to reduce your body weight. Those that follow a Mediterranean diet is able to help you to keep the weight off for a longer period of time as well.

Getting Started

Before we get started you have t understand the principles of the Mediterranean diet, and that's what this chapter is all about.

The principle behind Mediterranean dishes is natural, simple ingredients that can be found on the coast region. This leads to a variety of vegetables, fruit, whole grains, beans, healthy fats, red wine, beef, and fish. It's considered one of the healthiest diets.

Fruits & Vegetables

The first part of the Mediterranean diet is fresh fruits and vegetables. Most vegetable sand fruits are low in fat and high in fiber, which make them heart healthy. They can help with weight loss too.

They're also full of antioxidants which can help to reduce inflammation and slow down the aging process.

The antioxidants include vitamins A, vitamin C, vitamin E and vitamin K. they can help to remove harmful free radicals that can cause the oxidation of LDL, also known as bad cholesterol.

Whole Grains

This is also a must for the Mediterranean diet. Refined grains have been stripped of nutrients during the refinement process, which means they aren't as healthy as whole grains which have more nutrition. Whole grains have bran, endosperm and germ which are great for your health.

Some whole grain examples are brown rice, barley, bulgur, millet, oat, rye, teff, and wheat. Whole grains have quite a few benefits as well since they are more satisfying to your hunger and have phytochemicals which are disease-fighting chemicals.

Using Olive Oil

Olive oil has a lot of monounsaturated fats which can protect against heart disease because it keeps LDL levels, bad cholesterol, low and HDL levels, good cholesterol, high. Most Mediterranean meals are prepared by liberally using olive oil. Also, on the Mediterranean diet most foods are grilled or baked, which is easier to do with olive oil.

Fish & Chicken

The Mediterranean diet often includes and abundance of fresh fish because of the proximity of the area to the sea. Fish has a lot of omega-3 fatty acids which have various heart healthy benefits including reducing triglycerides, inflammation and even cholesterol. There are various types of fish to choose from as well, including salmon, mackerel, herring, sardines, trout and albacore tuna. Chicken can also be used in pace of fish to replace red meat. It isn't as healthy as fish, but it does have lower saturated fats and cholesterol than red meat.

Nuts

Unsalted nuts are often eaten as a snack in Mediterranean countries. However, the US is more likely to go for things such as crackers or potato chips which have no health benefits. Nuts can also be included in desserts and savory dishes. Pine nuts can be used to make homemade pesto, and you'll find walnuts are often in bread dough. Nuts are a wonderful source of monounsaturated fat, and they're packed full of protein and fiber. They can also contain various minerals and vitamins which will help to improve your overall health.

Red Wine

Small amounts of alcohol is consumed with most meals, especially red wine, in Mediterranean countries. It's been proven that alcoholic drinks, such as red win, have healthy heart benefits. Red wine has an antioxidant called flavonoids which can prevent fatty deposits from building up in the artery walls. Even the American Heart Association recommends one to two drinks a day for men and women. These drinks are only suppose to be four ounces each.

Spices

There are many spices and herbs that are used in the Mediterranean diet that also provide health benefits, including garlic. While these herbs and spices help to make the food taste great, their benefits to your health is the real magic.

The most common herbs and spices in this area are garlic, anise, basil, bay leaf, fennel, lavender, cumin, mint, marjoram, oregano, pepper, rosemary, sumaci, parsley, thyme and tarragon. Cutting down on salt can help to lower blood pressure, which is also a risk for heart disease, and these flavors help to lower your intake of salt. Garlic is a great way to spice up your meal, and you may not even know that the salt is missing!

Dairy

Full fat dairy products, including cheese and whole milk, are eaten in small amounts in Mediterranean countries. This helps to keep the saturated fat intake down. However, traditional cheeses such as goat cheese and feta cheese are lower in fat than hard cheeses such as Cheddar, which is extremely popular in the US. There is also yogurt which is eaten more frequently by being included in various dishes and desserts which is very healthy. Eggs can also be eaten regularly, but egg yolk is limited in this diet. Egg yolk should be limited to four per week to help to control your saturated fat intake. Though, egg whites can be eaten much more often.

Legumes

The importance of legumes is also emphasized in the Mediterranean diet. These include beans, peas, lentils and snap peas. Legumes have a high fiber and protein count which is a great addition to your diet.

Foods to Avoid

You should reduce red meat in the Mediterranean diet since it can contribute to heart disease, but you don't have to completely avoid it. With this diet, you don't have to completely avoid anything, but there are certain items that should be reduced and eaten sparingly. When you want to eat something like red meat, try to choose a small portion of lean red meat instead, and keep it down to three to four times per month. Here are some more foods to limit or avoid all together if possible.

- **Added Sugars:** This includes candies, ice cream, table sugar and soda.
- **Refined Grains:** This includes pasta that's made of refined wheat and white bread.
- **Trans Fat:** This can be found in various processed foods, but it's also in margarine!
- **Refined Oils:** This includes cottonseed oil, vegetable oil, canola oil and soybean oil.
- **Processed Meats:** Some common examples are processed hot dogs and sausages.
- **Highly Processed Foods:** This includes anything that is labeled "diet", "low fat" or was obviously made in a factory. Remember that you should be concentrating on whole, natural ingredients.

Swapping Food Out

If you're trying to stick to a Mediterranean diet, you need to know what common food you're eating can be swapped with to help keep you on track.

- **Butter:** Just swap it out for olive oil.

- **Salt:** Just swap it out for a variety of herbs and spices instead.
- **Mayonnaise:** Mayonnaise can be swapped out for mashed avocado.
- **Beer:** It's better to switch to a glass or two of red wine which has heart benefits.
- **Beef:** Beef isn't great for you, but you can usually swap it out for salmon which can easily be found at most grocery stores.
- **Potato Chips:** Instead of munching on something that has no health benefits, choose a bag of mixed nuts. Just make sure they're unsalted.
- **Jam or Jelly:** Swap it out for fresh fruit instead. You may want to even puree it in a food processor.
- **Rice or Bread:** While you can eat whole wheat bread and some rice on the Mediterranean diet, cut it back. If you're trying to cut back try to switch for legumes instead.
- **Cakes & Cookies:** Try vegetables and hummus for a healthy alternative that will curb your appetite.

The Take Away

Now that you know what you should and shouldn't eat, you need to make sure that you avoid as much temptation as possible. Clean out your home from things that are too unhealthy, especially at the beginning of your dietary change. It can be hard to stick to a lifestyle change. You'll also need to keep in mind your portion control, and you'll need to start making some time for physical activity even if it's just twenty minutes a day.

Top Tips

You already know that starting a new diet can be hard, and the Mediterranean diet is no different. Here are some top tips so that you can be successful with your dietary change.

When Dining Out

You aren't going to be able to stop going out to eat just because you're on a diet, especially when it's going to be a lifestyle change. Of course, you should try to limit dining out whenever possible for the first month of your lifestyle change. However, when you do go out to eat, start by dividing your meal in half. Don't wait either. You'll want to divide your plate the moment it comes to you. Save half for later, so ask for a take out container if at all possible. It's unlikely that you'll have food that fits your diet when eating out, so limiting your portion control is the first step in making sure you don't blow all of the hard work you've put in.

Never Skip Breakfast

When dieting, skipping a meal can seem like a good idea but it isn't. breakfast is one of the most commonly skipped meal because it's easier for you to wait for lunch than it is for someone to wait for dinner if they skip lunch. Though, skipping any meal can put your metabolism behind schedule. It's better to keep your refrigerator stocked with fruit and yogurt for small, light breakfasts that are also great on the go.

Chop Your Vegetables

It's best to chop your vegetables in advance so that you can use them for snacks and quick lunches. Some of the best vegetables to keep on hand for this is bell peppers, celery, carrots and cucumbers. They're also perfect for dipping in hummus which is a healthy snack too!

Shop Locally

You may want to pay a visit to your local farmer's market as well. It's a great way to keep your house stocked full with seasonal vegetables that are sure to be fresh. It can also help to cut costs if you're shopping locally and seasonally. You shouldn't let your budget be your downfall when making an important lifestyle change, and shopping locally sourced food can help.

Keep Nuts & Seeds

It's just as important that you keep nuts and seeds on hand for a healthy alternative to chips, cookies and other processed foods. Some great choices are sunflower seeds, almonds or walnuts. Remember that these shouldn't be salted either!

Use Fruit More

You can use fruit for dessert and even add some sweetness by drizzling honey or brown sugar over the top. Fresh fruit is a healthy snack when your stomach is hungry too, but the added, healthy sweetener should only be used when using it for dessert.

Eat Slower

You should savor your food if you want to make sure you aren't rushing through and eating more than you need to. If you cherish your time eating by sharing it with family and friends you will eat slower and consume less calories. You're also more likely to want to put in the extra effort to make a healthy, tasty meal which make take some time. That's why getting your family involved is also a healthful tip.

Use Whole Grains

You already know that whole grains are an essential part of the Mediterranean diet, so you need to switch to them for success. Minimally processed grains are healthier including couscous, bulgur, barley, oats rice, polenta, faro and millet.

Manage Portions

The Mediterranean diet encourages portion control. Don't concentrate on counting calories. Instead, you need to concentrate on the quality of calories that you're eating. Calories are important, but your calorie type is much more important. This diet has nutrient dense food that will help you to stay full in the long run, so you don't have to eat a large amount of it. Always keep an eye on your plate size if you want to stay on track.

Some Kitchen Staples

You already know the basics of what you should and shouldn't eat. In this chapter we'll go over some kitchen staples you can keep on hand to help improve the chances of success on your diet.

Almonds

Almonds have a lot of health benefits, including their ability to promote weight loss and lower cholesterol. They're best when consumed raw, but they're also frequently used in Mediterranean dishes.

Couscous

This is a whole grain that has a lot of fiber, antioxidant phytochemicals, magnesium, and vitamin E. Couscous is digested slowly which can help to prevent spikes in insulin and glucose, which can help to protect you against diabetes, disease and other chronic diseases. It can be used as aside dish for beans or fish, and it can be added to salad easily.

Tomatoes

Tomatoes are packed with lycopene which is an antioxidant that helps to prevent some cancers. They're also full of vitamin C, and they're versatile too. You can use them fresh, canned or even in paste form. They're budget friendly too!

Yogurt

You need intestinal bacteria to keep your body moving smoothly, which yogurt is great at cultivating. It also contains vitamin B2, vitamin B12, potassium, calcium and magnesium. Yogurt can be used for salad dressings too. Just choose a low fat yogurt that doesn't have a lot of added sugar.

Chickpeas

These are healthy and filling, and they contain a lot of fiber too. Fiber helps to prevent colon cancer, reduce heart disease risk and manage diabetes. When combined with grains and starches, they add high protein value along with calcium, iron, folate and zinc.

Olive Oil

This has a high amount of monounsaturated fatty acids which are great for you. You should choose high quality extra virgin olive oil because the oil is collected through cold pressing. This removes the oil under pressure without the use of heat, which means it's keeping the antioxidants and monounsaturated fat that's healthy for you. You can even use olive oil after cooking to add a little extra flavor to your meal by drizzling it over bread, pasta or vegetables.

Rice

This is a carb that gives your body the energy it needs. It helps to improve and regulates bowel movements and stabilize your blood sugars. It provides instant energy, and it's a great side dish when portion controlled.

It can also be used in different ways, so it doesn't have to be routine or boring. You can cook it with fish, lentils, beans, vegetables, meats and spices.

Eggplant

This is another vegetable that you'll want to keep on hand for fiber, potassium and chlorogenic acid which is found in the eggplant skin. This is an antiviral and it can help to fight cancer. There are several methods you can cook eggplant with including broiling, baking, stir frying, frying, roasting, and even grilling.

Garlic

Garlic will help your immune system because it contains a large dose of vitamin C and antioxidants. It's a seasoning that's versatile and works well in savory dishes. It can be used in salad dressing, soups, stews, sauces, bread, grain dishes and even casseroles.

Lentils

These are packed with B vitamins, protein, fiber and phytochemicals. They're also economical, which will help your budget stretch a little further. They create a great texture and flavor for your meal, and you don't have to soak them before you start cooking like with beans.

All you have to do is sort them, discarding any dirty or discolored ones, rinse them, and cook them according to your recipe or package instructions.

Breakfast Recipes

Spinach Omelet

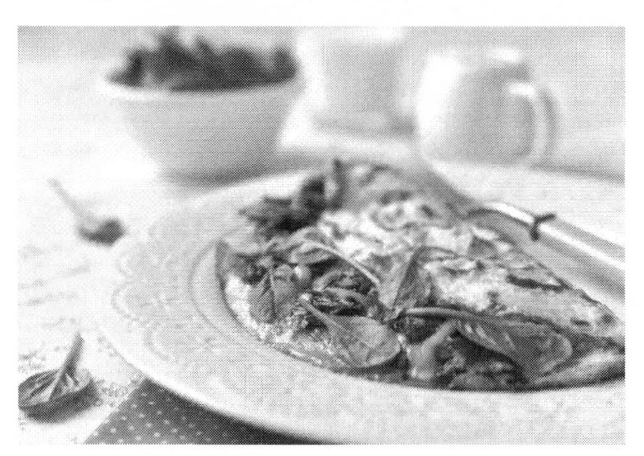

Serves: 4
Time: 30 Minutes
Calories: 295
Protein: 15 Grams
Fat: 23 Grams
Carbs: 10 Grams
Ingredients:

- 3 Tablespoons Olive Oil
- 1 Onion, Small & Chopped
- 1 Clove Garlic, Minced
- 4 Tomatoes, Large, Cored & Chopped
- 1 Teaspoon Sea Salt, Fine
- 8 Eggs, Beaten
- ¼ Teaspoon Black Pepper
- 2 Ounces Feta cheese, Crumbled
- 1 Tablespoon Flat Leaf Parsley, Fresh & Chopped

Directions:

1. Start by heating your oven to 400, and then place your olive oil in an ovenproof skillet. Place your skillet over high heat, adding in your onions. Cook for five to seven minutes. Your onions should soften.
2. Add your tomatoes, salt, pepper and garlic in. simmer for another five minutes, and then pour in your beaten eggs. Mix lightly, and cook for three to five minutes. They should set at the bottom. Put the pan in the oven, baking for five minutes more.
3. Remove from the oven, topping with parsley and feta. Serve warm.

Mango Pear Smoothie

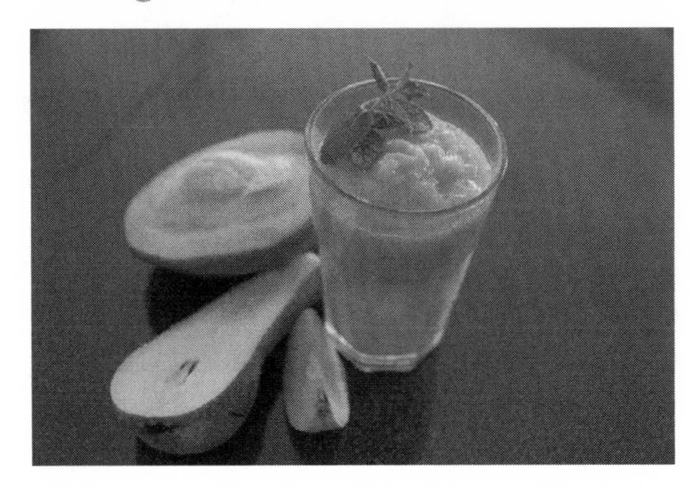

Serves: 1
Time: 10 Minutes
Calories: 293
Protein: 8 Grams
Fa: 8 Grams
Carbs: 53 Grams
Ingredients:

- 2 Ice Cubes
- ½ Cup Greek Yogurt, Plain
- ½ Mango, Peeled, Pitted & Chopped
- 1 Cup Kale, Chopped
- 1 Pear, Ripe, Cored & Chopped

Directions:

1. Blend together until thick and smooth. Serve chilled.

Quinoa Fruit Salad

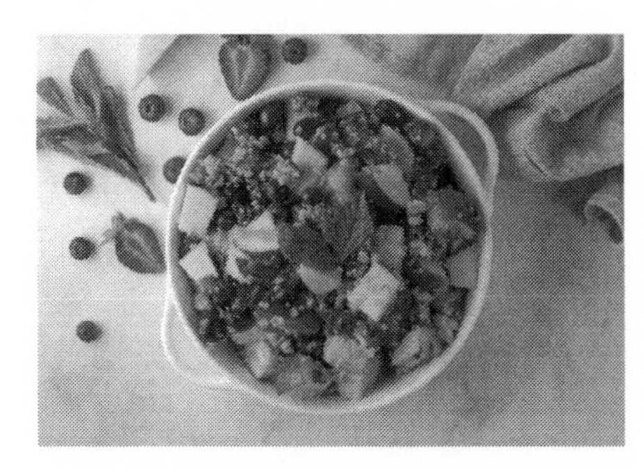

Serves: 4
Time: 25 Minutes
Calories: 206
Protein: 5 Grams
Fat: 2 Grams
Carbs: 45 Grams
Ingredients:

- 2 Tablespoons Honey, Raw
- 1 Cup Strawberries, Fresh & Sliced
- 2 Tablespoons Lime Juice, Fresh
- 1 Teaspoon Basil, Fresh & Chopped
- 1 Cup Quinoa, Cooked
- 1 Mango, Peeled, Pitted & Diced
- 1 Cup Blackberries, Fresh
- 1 Peach, Pitted & Diced
- 2 Kiwis, Peeled & Quartered

Directions:

1. Start by mixing your lime juice, basil and honey together in a small bowl.
2. In a different bowl mix your strawberries, quinoa, blackberries, peach, kiwis and mango. Add in your honey mixture, and toss to coat before serving.

Almond Pancakes

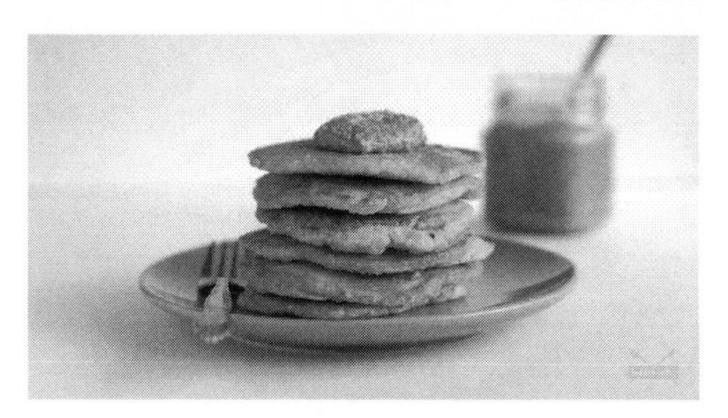

Serves: 6
Time: 30 Minutes
Calories: 286
Protein: 6 Grams
Fat: 17 Grams
Carbs: 27 Gram
Ingredients:

- 2 Cups Almond Milk, Unsweetened & Room Temperature
- 2 Eggs, Large & Room Temperature
- ½ Cup Coconut Oil, Melted + More for Greasing
- 2 Teaspoons Honey, Raw
- ¼ Teaspoon Sea Salt, Fine
- ½ Teaspoon Baking Soda
- 1 ½ Cups Whole Wheat Flour
- ½ Cup Almond Flour
- 1 ½ Teaspoons Baking Powder
- ¼ Teaspoon Cinnamon, Ground

Directions:

1. Get out a large bowl and whisk your coconut oil, eggs, almond milk and honey, blending until it's mixed well.

2. Get a medium bowl out and sift together your baking powder, baking soda, almond flour, sea salt, whole wheat flour and cinnamon. Mix well.
3. Add your flour mixture to your milk mixture, and whisk well.
4. Get out a large skillet and grease it using your coconut oil before placing it over medium-high heat. Add in your pancake batter in ½ cup measurements.
5. Cook for three minutes or until the edges are firm. The bottom of your pancake should be golden, and bubbles should break the surface. Flip and cook for two minutes on the other side. They should be cooked all the way through, and then get out a plate to put them on.
6. Wipe your skillet with a clean paper towel, and repeat until all of your batter is used. Make sure to re-grease your skillet, and top with fresh fruit if desired.

Strawberry Rhubarb Smoothie

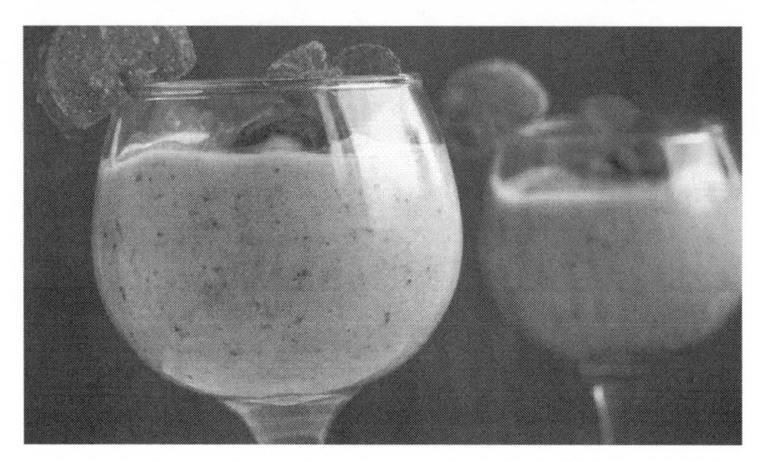

Serves: 1
Time: 8 Minutes
Calories: 295
Protein: 6 Grams
Fat: 8 Grams
Carbs: 56 Grams
Ingredients:

- 1 Cup Strawberries, Fresh & Sliced
- 1 Rhubarb Stalk, Chopped
- 2 Tablespoons Honey, Raw
- 3 Ice Cubes
- 1/8 Teaspoon Ground Cinnamon
- ½ Cup Greek Yogurt, Plain

Directions:

1. Start by getting out a small saucepan and fill it with water. Place it over high heat to bring it to a boil, and then add in your rhubarb. Boil for three minutes before draining and transferring it to a blender.

2. In your blender add in your yogurt, honey, cinnamon and strawberries. Blend until smooth, and then add in your ice. Blend until there are no lumps and it's thick. Enjoy cold.

Bircher Muesli

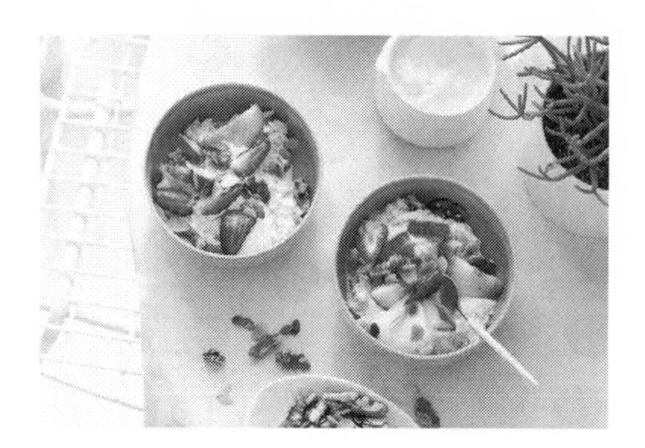

Serves: 4
Time: 6 Hours 10 Minutes
Calories: 397
Protein: 9 Grams
Fat: 18 Grams
Carbs: 55 Grams
Ingredients:

- 1 ½ Cup Rolled Oats
- ½ Cup Coconut, Unsweetened & Shredded
- 2 Cups Almond Milk, Unsweetened
- 2 Bananas, Mashed
- ½ Cup Raisins
- ½ Cup Almonds, Chopped
- ½ Teaspoon Cinnamon, Ground

Directions:

1. Get out a large container that is able to be sealed and stir together your coconut, oats and almond milk. Make sure that it's well mixed, and then allow it to soak for six hours or overnight.
2. Stir in your almonds, raisins, banana and cinnamon before serving chilled.

Gingerbread & Pumpkin Smoothie

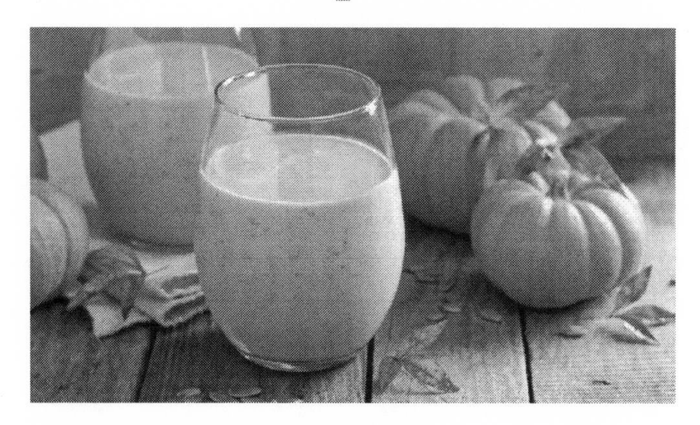

Serves: 1
Time: 1 Hour 5 Minutes
Calories: 200
Fat: 5 Grams
Carbs: 41 Grams
Ingredients:

- 1 Cup Almond Milk, Unsweetened
- 2 Teaspoons Chia Seeds
- 1 Banana
- ½ Cup Pumpkin Puree, Canned
- ¼ Teaspoon Ginger, Ground
- ¼ Teaspoon Cinnamon, Ground
- 1/8 Teaspoon Nutmeg, Ground

Directions:

1. Start by getting out a bowl and mix your chai seeds and almond milk. Allow them to soak for at least an hour, but you can soak them overnight. Transfer them to a blender.
2. Add in your remaining ingredients, and then blend until smooth. Serve chilled.

Barley Porridge

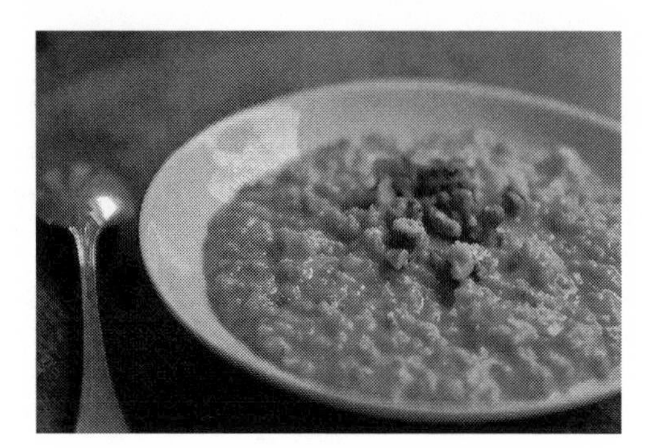

Serves: 4
Time: 30 Minutes
Calories: 354
Protein: 11 Grams
Fat: 8 Grams
Carbs: 63 Grams
Ingredients:

- 1 Cup Wheat Berries
- 1 Cup Barley
- 2 Cups Almond Milk, Unsweetened + More for Serving
- ½ Cup Blueberries
- ½ Cup Pomegranate Seeds
- 2 Cups Water
- ½ Cup Hazelnuts, Toasted & Chopped
- ¼ Cup Honey, Raw

Directions:

1. Get out a saucepan and put it over medium-high heat, and then add in your almond milk, water, barley and wheat berries. Bring it to a boil before reducing the heat to low, and allow it to simmer for twenty-five minutes. Stir frequently. Your grains should become tender.

2. Top each serving with blueberries, pomegranate seeds, hazelnuts, a tablespoon of honey and a splash of almond milk.

Walnut & Date Smoothie

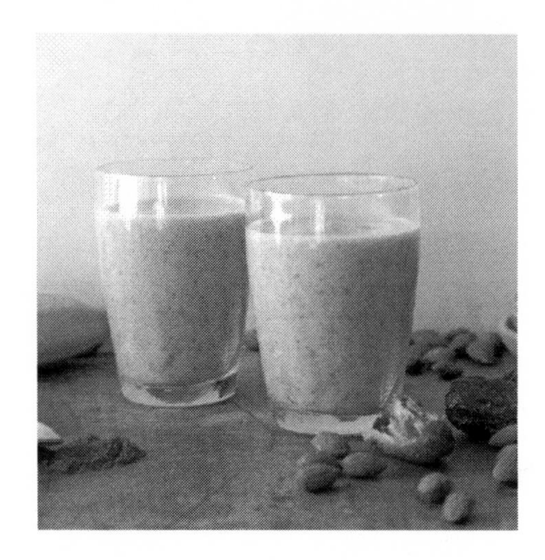

Serves: 2
Time: 10 Minutes
Calories: 385
Protein: 21 Grams
Fat: 17 Grams
Carbs: 35 Grams
Ingredients:

- 4 Dates, Pitted
- ½ Cup Milk
- 2 Cups Greek Yogurt, Plain
- 1/2 Cup Walnuts
- ½ Teaspoon Cinnamon, Ground
- ½ Teaspoon Vanilla Extract, Pure
- 2-3 Ice Cubes

Directions:

1. Blend everything together until smooth, and then serve chilled.

Lunch Recipes

Chicken & Rice Soup

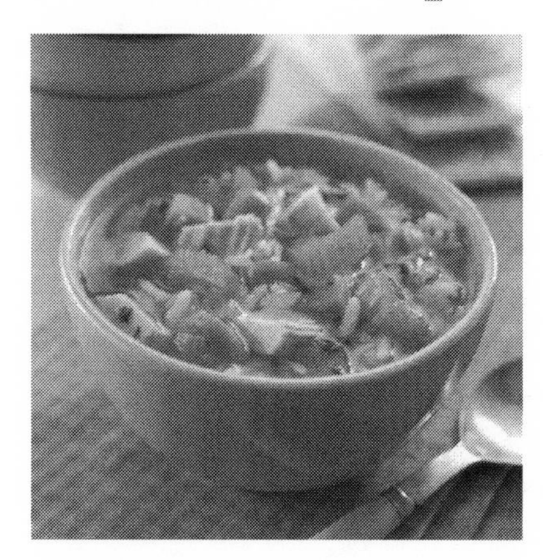

Serves: 4
Time: 35 Minutes
Calories: 382
Protein: 27 Grams
Fat: 15 Grams
Carbs: 34 Grams
Ingredients:

- 1/4 Cup Olive oil
- 2 Leeks, Root & Tops Trimmed, Sliced Thin
- 1 Fennel Bulb, Chopped
- 2 Carrots, Peeled & Sliced Thin
- 1 Clove Garlic, Sliced
- ½ Cup Rice
- 6 Cups Chicken Broth
- 1 Teaspoon Sea Salt, Fine
- ¼ Teaspoon Black Pepper
- 2 Sprigs Thyme, Fresh
- 2 Cups Chicken, Cooked & Cut into ½ Inch Cubes

- 1 Lemon, Zested & Juiced
- 2 Scallions, Sliced Thin

Directions:

1. Heat your olive oil in a Dutch oven, and then add in your garlic, carrot, fennel and leeks. Sauté until your vegetables are lightly browned. Add in your rice, stirring well.
2. add in your thyme, slat, pepper and chicken broth. Bring it t o a boil before reducing it to a simmer. Cook while covered for fifteen minutes. The rice should become tender.
3. Add in your lemon juice, lemon zest, scallions and chicken. Remove the thyme, and serve warm.

Mushroom Risotto

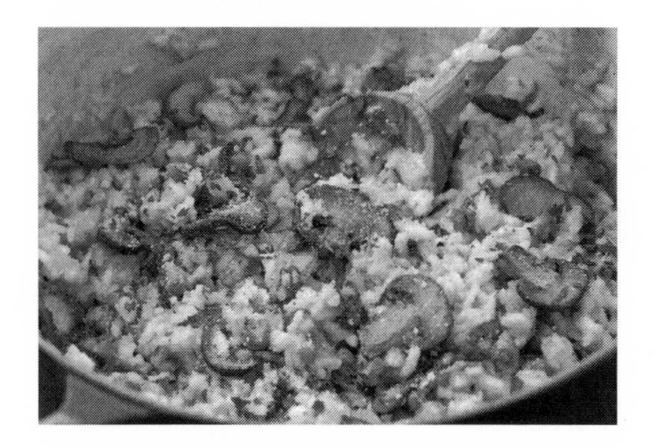

Serves: 4
Time: 40 Minutes
Calories: 322
Protein: 14 Grams
Fat: 11 Grams
Carbs: 38 Grams
Ingredients:

- 2 Tablespoons Olive Oil
- 1 Shallot, Sliced Thin
- 10 Mushrooms, Large & Sliced
- ½ Cup Red Wine
- 1 Cup Faro
- ½ Cup Vegetable Broth
- ½ Cup Parmesan Cheese
- 1 Tablespoon Flatleaf Parsley, Fresh & Chopped
- ¼ Teaspoon Black Pepper
- 1 Teaspoon Sea Salt, Fine

Directions:

1. Place a skillet over high heat, adding in your shallot and olive oil. Cook for three to five minutes. It should soften, and then add in your red wine and mushrooms. Cook until the wine has evaporated.
2. Add in your faro, cooking for three minutes. Coat it, and then add in ½ cup broth. Stir occasionally while cooking. Your broth should be absorbed, and then add another half a cup. Continue to repeat, and the faro should be tender but not mushy.
3. Turn the heat off, adding in your parsley, salt, pepper and parmesan. Serve warm.

Sun Dried Tomato Quiche

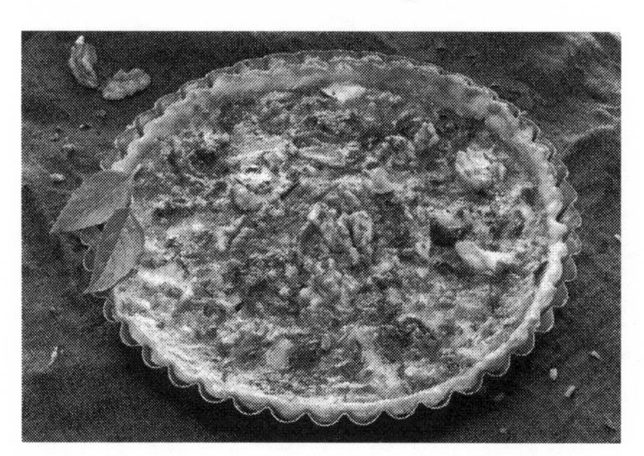

Serves: 4
Time: 40 Minutes
Calories: 171
Protein: 13 Grams
Fat: 11 Grams
Carbs: 5 Grams
Ingredients:

- 6 Eggs, Large
- ¼ Cup Goat Cheese
- 1/8 Teaspoon Cayenne Pepper
- 2 Tablespoons Milk
- 2 Shallots, Chopped Fine
- 1 Teaspoon Olive Oil
- ½ Teaspoon Garlic, Minced
- 1 Teaspoon Parsley, Fresh & Chopped
- ¼ Teaspoon Sea Salt, Fine
- ¼ Teaspoon Black Pepper
- 10 Sun Dried Tomatoes, Quartered

Directions:

1. Start by heating your oven to 375, and then get out a bowl. Whisk your goat cheese, milk, cayenne and eggs together until they're well blended.

2. Get out an ovenproof skillet that's nine inches, and place it over medium-high heat. Add in your olive oil.
3. Once your olive oil is hot add in your garlic and shallots, and sauté for two minutes. They should be tender and fragrant.
4. Pour your egg mix in, and then scatter your sun dried tomatoes and parsley on top.
5. Season with salt and pepper, and cook it while lifting the edges so that the uncooked egg flows underneath. It will take about three minutes for the bottom to firm.
6. Put your skillet in the oven, and bake for twenty minutes. It should be golden, puffy and the egg should be cooked all the way through.

Artichoke Frittata

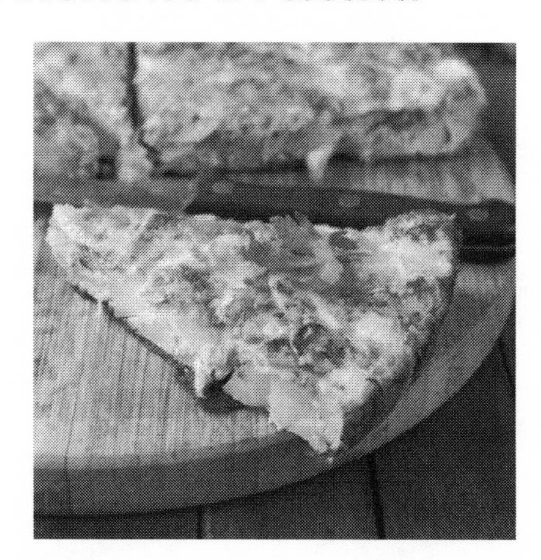

Serves: 4
Time: 15 Minutes
Calories; 199
Protein: 16 Grams
Fat: 13 Grams
Carbs: 5 Grams
Ingredients:

- 8 Eggs, Large
- ¼ Cup Asiago Cheese, Grated
- 1 Tablespoon Basil, Fresh & Chopped
- 1 Teaspoon Oregano, Fresh & Chopped
- ¼ Teaspoon Sea Salt, Fine
- ¼ Teaspoon Black Pepper
- 1 Teaspoon Olive Oil
- 1 Teaspoon Garlic, Minced
- 1 Can Water Packed Artichoke Hearts, Quartered & Drained
- 1 Tomato, Chopped

Directions:

1. Start by heating your oven to a broil, and then get out a bowl. Whisk your asiago cheese, basil, oregano, eggs, pepper and salt together. Make sure it's well blended, and then get out a skillet that's ovenproof. Place it over medium-high heat, and heat up your olive oil. Add in your garlic and sauté for a minute.
2. Remove it from the skillet, and then heat and pour in your egg mixture. Return the skillet to heat before sprinkling in your tomato and artichoke hearts.
3. Cook without stirring for eight minutes. The center should set. Place your skillet in the oven, and broil for a minute. The top should be puffed and lightly brown.
4. Serve warm.

Eggplant Soup

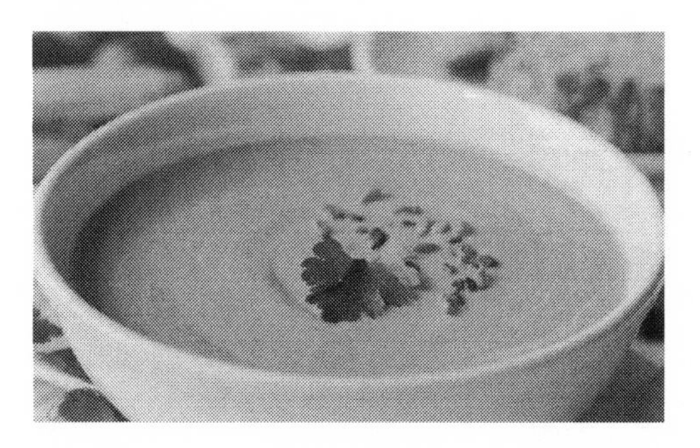

Serves: 4
Time: 1 Hour 30 Minutes
Calories: 294
Protein: 8 Grams
Fat: 17 Grams
Carbs: 33 Grams
Ingredients:

- 2 Eggplants, Halved
- 1 Teaspoon Sea Salt, Fine
- 2 Teaspoon Cumin, Ground
- 1 Teaspoon Coriander, Ground
- 1 Tablespoon Olive Oil
- 1 Sweet Onion, Peeled & Diced
- 4 Cups Vegetable Stock
- 1 Tablespoon Garlic, Minced
- ½ Cup Heavy Whipping Cream
- ¼ Cup Tahini
- 1 Tablespoon Cilantro, Fresh & Chopped

Directions:

1. Sprinkle your eggplant with sea salt, and set it to the side for a half hour. Preheat your oven to 400.

2. Rinse your eggplant and then place them on the baking sheet with the cut side down. Roast it of a half hour. It should be soft and collapsed, and then scoop out the flesh, placing it in the large bowl. Set it to the side, and then get out a large stockpot.
3. Place your stockpot over medium-high heat, and then heat the olive oil. Add the garlic and onion, and sauté for three minutes. It should be softened.
4. Add in your cumin, coriander, vegetable stock, and eggplant flesh. Allow the mixture to bring it to a boil and then reduce the heat to low. Let it simmer for ten minutes, but stir frequently.
5. Get a handheld immersion blender and puree until smooth.
6. Stir in your tahini and heavy cream, and then sere warm. Garnish with cilantro.

Cucumber Salad

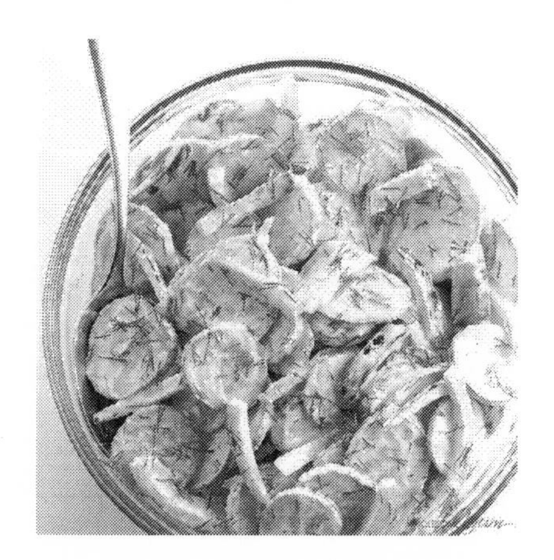

Serves: 4
Time: 10 Minutes
Calories: 68
Protein: 4 Grams
Fat: 1 Gram
Carbs: 11 Grams
Ingredients:

- 5-6 Cucumbers, Small, Peeled & Diced
- 8 Ounces Greek Yogurt, Plain
- 2 Cloves Garlic, Minced
- 1 Teaspoon Oregano
- 1 Tablespoon Mint, Fresh & Minced
- 1/8 Teaspoon Sea Salt, Fine
- 1/8 Teaspoon Black Pepper

Directions:

1. Get out cucumbers, yogurt, garlic, mint and oregano, mixing them in a large bowl. Season with salt and pepper, and then refrigerate for an hour before serving.

Goat Cheese Salad

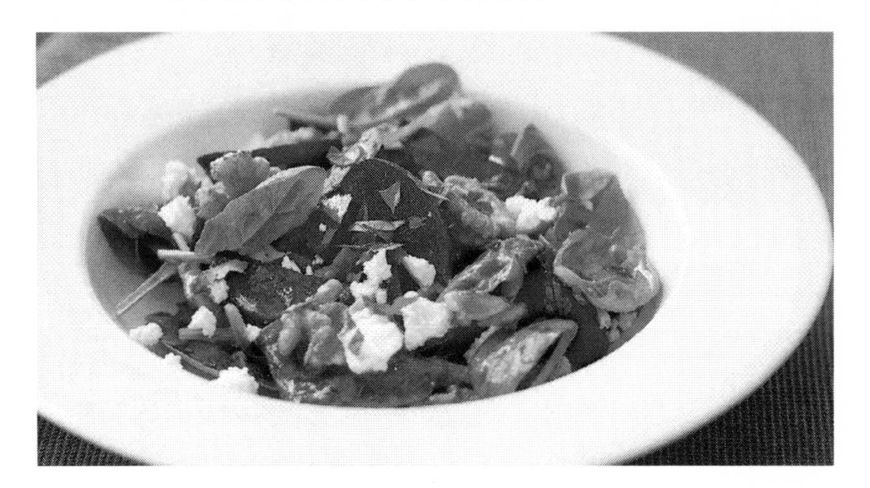

Serves: 4
Time: 35 Minutes
Calories: 322
Protein: 18 Grams
Fat: 11 Grams
Carbs: 35 Grams
Ingredients:

- 1 Head Garlic
- Olive Oil as Needed for Drizzling
- 1/4 Teaspoon Sea Salt, Fine
- 1/4 Teaspoon Black Pepper
- 2 Teaspoons Basil, Fresh & Chopped
- 4 Ounces Goat Cheese, Room Temperature
- 8 Slices Whole Wheat Bread
- 2 Cups Spinach, Fresh & Shredded
- 2 Roasted Red Bell Peppers, Halved, Seed & Cut into Strips

Directions:

1. Start by heating your oven to 350, and then slice off the top of your garlic head. Once the cloves are exposed, drizzle them with olive oil before placing

them in a baking dish. Roast them of twenty to twenty-five minutes. The cloves should be soft and fragrant. Them to the side and allow them to cool.

2. Get out a bowl and stir your basil, goat cheese, a teaspoon of roasted garlic, salt and pepper together until it makes a soft mixture.
3. Toast your bread, and lightly spread the goat cheese mixture across it. Top each slice with a quarter of roasted peppers, and then heap about a half a cup of spinach on each sandwich. Put your slices together to make a sandwich and serve.

Chicken & Vegetable Wraps

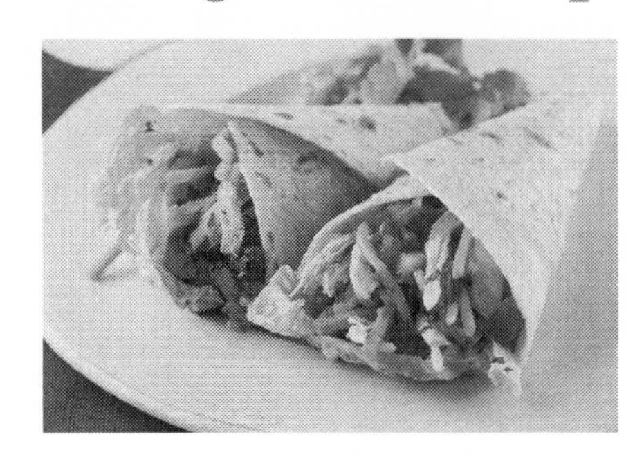

Serves: 4
Time: 15 Minutes
Calories: 278
Protein: 27 Grams
Fat: 7 Grams
Carbs: 28 Grams
Ingredients:

- ¼ Cup Greek Yogurt, Plain
- 2 Cups Chicken, Cooked & Chopped
- ½ Red Bell Pepper, Diced
- ½ English Cucumber, Diced
- ½ Cup Carrot, Shredded
- 1 Scallion, Chopped
- ½ Teaspoon Thyme, Fresh & Chopped
- 1 Tablespoon Lemon Juice, Fresh
- 4 Tortillas, Multigrain
- ¼ Teaspoon Sea Salt, Fine
- ¼ Teaspoon Black Pepper

Directions:

1. Start by getting out a bowl and mix your cucumber, red bell pepper, chicken, scallion, carrot, lemon juice, thyme, yogurt, sea salt and pepper. Mix well.

2. Spoon a quarter of this mixture into each tortilla, folding it over to make a pocket. Repeat with your remaining ingredients.

Snack Recipes

Sweet & Sour Pumpkin Mix

Serves: 4
Time: 45 Minutes
Calories: 301
Protein: 5 Grams
Fat: 19 Grams
Carbs: 34 Grams
Ingredients:

- ¼ Cup Olive Oil
- 4 Cups Pumpkin, Peeled & Seeded, Cut into 1 Inch Cubes
- ½ Teaspoon Black Pepper
- 1 Teaspoon Sea Salt, Fine
- 2 Teaspoons Honey, Raw
- 2 Teaspoons Red Wine Vinegar
- 1 Onion, Large & Sliced Thin
- 1 Teaspoon Cinnamon, Ground
- ¼ Cup Raisins
- ¼ Cup Pine Nuts, Toasted

Directions:

1. Get out a Dutch oven and add in your onion and olive oil. Sauté until the omens are tender, which should take roughly five minutes. Add in your pumpkin, and cook for five minutes over medium heat.
2. Add in your salt, pepper, vinegar, cinnamon, sugar, and raisins. Cover, cooking on low heat for twenty minutes. The squash should become tender, and you'll need to stir occasionally.

3. Spoon your pumpkin into a serving dish, and sprinkle with pine nuts to serve.

Sautéed Apricots

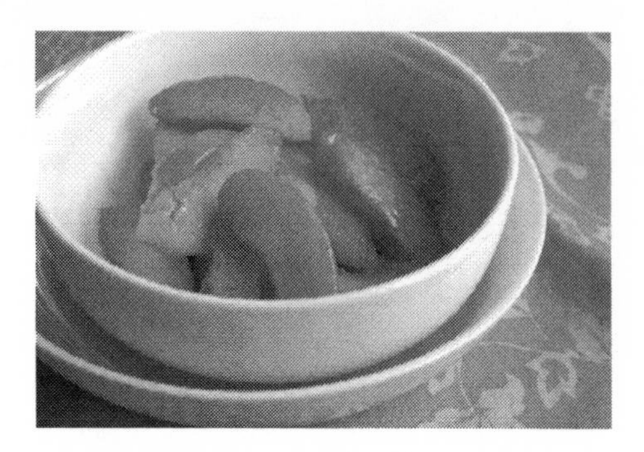

Serves: 4
Time: 15 Minutes
Calories: 207
Protein: 5 Grams
Fat: 19 Grams
Carbs: 7 Grams
Ingredients:

- 2 Tablespoons Olive Oil
- 1 Cup Almonds, Blanched, Skinless & Unsalted
- ½ Teaspoon Sea Salt, Fine
- 1/8 Teaspoon Red Pepper Flakes
- 1/8 Teaspoon Cinnamon, Ground
- ½ Cup Apricots, Dried & Chopped

Directions:

1. Place a frying pan over high heat, adding in your almonds, salt and olive oil. Sauté until the almonds turn a light gold, which will take five to ten minutes. Make sure to stir often because they burn easily.
2. Spoon your almonds into a serving dish, adding in your cinnamon, red pepper flakes, and chopped apricot.
3. Allow it to cool before serving.

Spiced Kale Chips

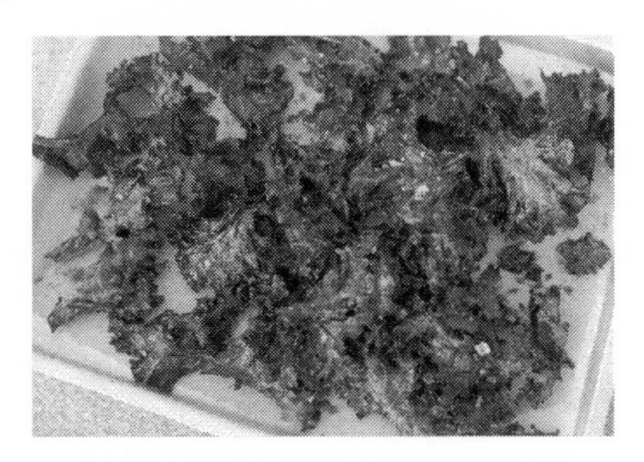

Serves: 4
Time: 35 Minutes
Calories: 56
Protein: 2 Grams
Fat: 4 Grams
Carbs: 5 Grams
Ingredients:

- 1 Tablespoon Olive Oil
- ½ Teaspoon Chili Powder
- ¼ Teaspoon Sea Salt, Fine
- 3 Cups Kale, Stemmed, Washed & Torn into 2 Inch Pieces

Directions:

1. Start by heating your oven to 300, and then get out two baking sheets. Line each baking sheet with parchment paper before placing them to the side.
2. Dry your kale off completely before placing it in a bowl, and add in your olive oil. Make sure the kale is thoroughly coated before seasoning it.
3. Spread your kale out on your baking sheets in a single layer, baking for twenty-five minutes. Your kale will need roasted halfway through, and it should turn out dry and crispy.
4. Allow them to cool for at least five minutes before serving.

Yogurt Dip

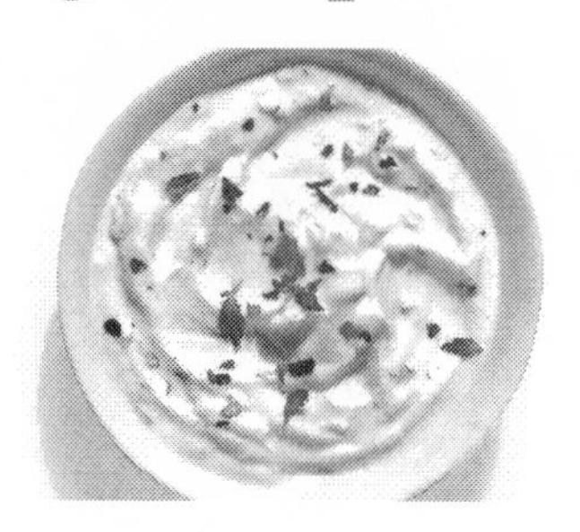

Serves: 4
Time: 10 Minutes
Calories: 59
Protein: 2 Grams
Fat: 4 Grams
Carbs: 5 Grams
Ingredients:

- ½ Lemon, Juiced & Zested
- 1 Cup Greek Yogurt, Plain
- 1 Tablespoon Chives, Fresh & Chopped Fine
- 2 Teaspoons Dill, Fresh & Chopped
- 2 Teaspoons Thyme, Fresh & Chopped
- 1 Teaspoon Parsley, Fresh & Chopped
- ½ Teaspoon Garlic, Minced
- ¼ Teaspoon Sea Salt, Fine

Directions:

1. Get out a bowl and mix all of your ingredients together until they're well blended. Season with salt before refrigerating. Serve chilled.

Zucchini Fritters

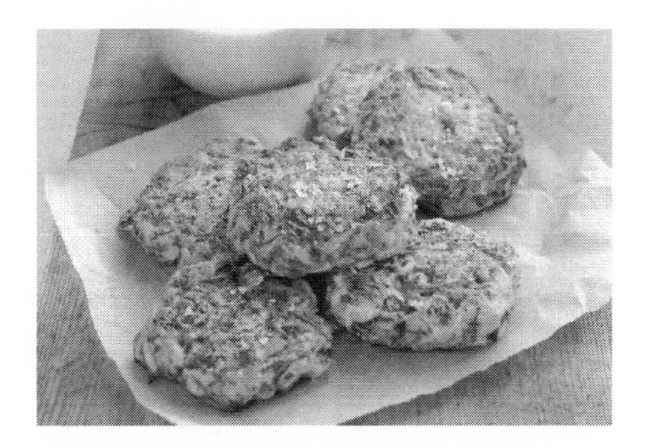

Serves: 6
Time: 30 Minutes
Calories: 103
Protein: 5 Grams
Fat: 8 Grams
Carbs: 5 Grams
Ingredients:

- 2 Zucchinis, Peeled & Grated
- 1 Sweet Onion, Diced Fine
- 2 Cloves Garlic, Minced
- 1 Cup Parsley, Fresh & Chopped
- ½ Teaspoon Sea Salt, Fine
- ½ Teaspoon Black Pepper
- ½ Teaspoon Allspice, Ground
- 2 Tablespoons Olive Oil
- 4 Eggs, Large

Directions:

1. Get out a plate and line it with paper towels before setting it to the side.
2. Get out a large bowl and mix your onion, parsley, garlic, zucchini, pepper, allspice and sea salt together.

3. Get out a different bowl and beat your eggs before adding them to your zucchini mixture. Make sure it's mixed well.
4. Get out a large skillet and place it over medium heat. Heat up your olive oil, and then scoop ¼ cup at a time into the skillet to create your fritters. Cook for three minutes or until the bottom sets. Flip and cook for an additional three minutes. Transfer them to your plate so they can drain. Serve with pita bread or on their own.

Easy Hummus

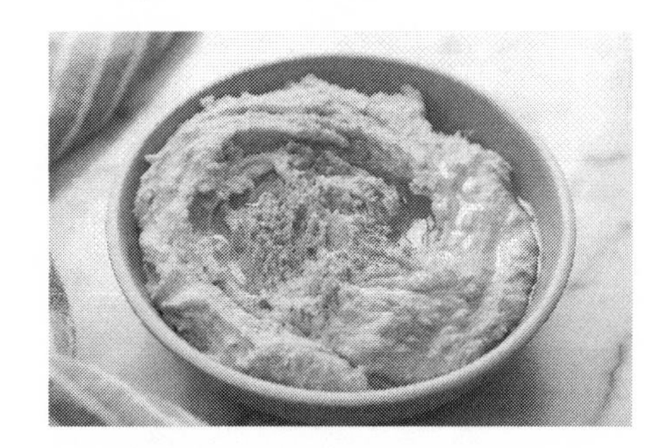

Serves: 6
Time: 5 Minutes
Calories: 187
Protein: 8 Gram
Fat: 7 Grams
Carbs: 25 Grams
Ingredients:

- 3 Cloves Garlic, Crushed
- 1 Tablespoon Olive Oil
- 1 Teaspoon Sea Salt, Fine
- 16 Ounces Canned Garbanzo Beans, Drained
- 1 ½ Tablespoons Tahini
- ½ Cup Lemon Juice, Fresh

Directions:

1. Blend your garbanzo beans, tahini, garlic, olive oil, lemon juice and sea salt together for three to five minutes in a blender. Make sure it's mixed well. It should be fluffy and soft.
2. Refrigerate for at least an hour before serving with either pita bread or cut vegetables.

Dinner Recipes

Tomato Linguine

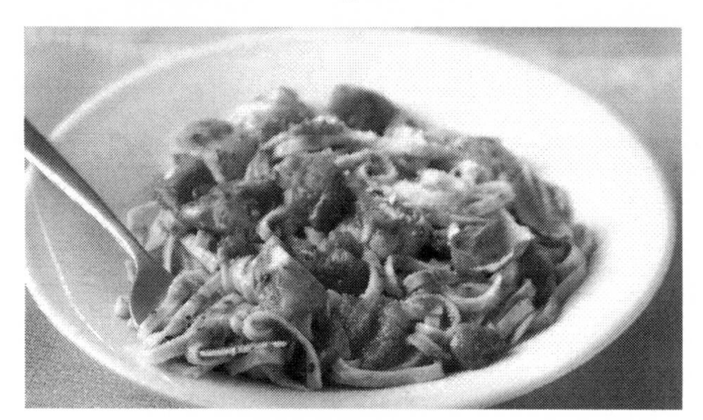

Serves: 4
Time: 25 Minutes
Calories: 397
Protein: 13 Grams
Fat: 15 Grams
Carbs: 55 Grams
Ingredients:

- 2 lb. Cherry Tomatoes
- 2 Tablespoons Balsamic Vinegar
- 3 Tablespoons Olive Oil
- 2 Teaspoons Garlic, Minced
- ¾ lb. Linguine Pasta, Whole Wheat
- ¼ Teaspoon black Pepper
- ¼ Cup Feta Cheese, Crumbled
- 1 Tablespoon Oregano, Fresh & Chopped

Directions:

1. Start by heating your oven to 350, and then get out a baking sheet. Line your baking sheet with parchment paper before setting it aside.

2. Get out a bowl and then toss two tablespoons of olive oil, garlic, balsamic vinegar, pepper and tomatoes together until well coated. Spread your tomatoes on your baking sheet, roasting for fifteen minutes. They should soften and burst open.
3. Cook your pasta according to package directions, and then drain it, placing it in a bowl.
4. Toss your pasta with the remaining olive oil and add in your tomatoes.
5. Serve topped with feta and oregano.

Asparagus & Kale Pesto Pasta

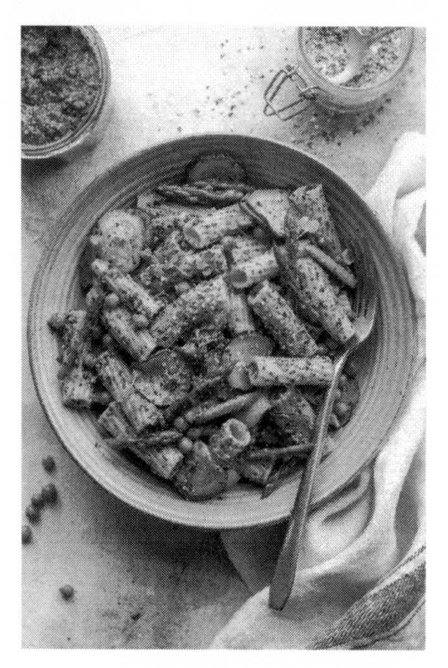

Serves: 6
Time: 20 Minutes
Calories: 283
Protein: 10 Grams
Fat: 12 Grams
Carbs: 33 Grams
Ingredients:

- ¼ Cup Basil, Fresh
- ¾ lb. Asparagus, Trimmed & Chopped Roughly
- ¼ lb. Kale, Washed
- ½ Cup Asiago Cheese, Grated
- ¼ Cup Olive Oil
- 1 Lemon, Juiced & Zested
- ¼ Teaspoon Sea Salt, Fine
- ¼ Teaspoon Black Pepper

- 1 lb. Angel Hair Pasta

Directions:

1. Start by pulsing your kale and asparagus in a food processor until it's finely chopped. Add in your olive oil, lemon juice, basil, and asiago cheese. Continue to pulse until it forms a pesto that's smooth, seasoning with salt and pepper.
2. Cook your pasta according to package instructions before draining it and placing it in a bowl.
3. Add in your pesto and make sure to toss to coat. Sprinkle with lemon zest before serving.

Vegetarian Lasagna

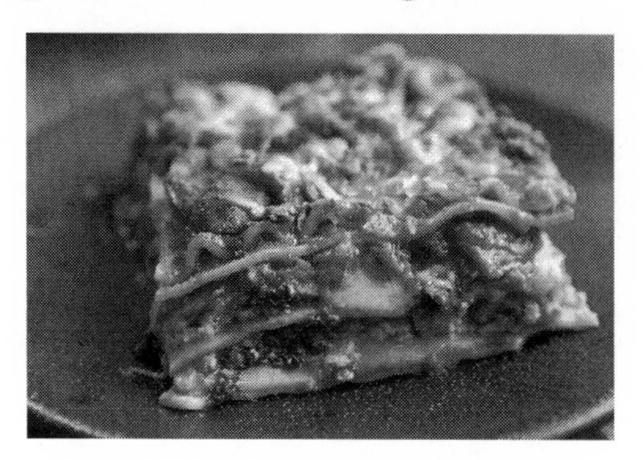

Serves: 6
Time: 1 Hour 15 Minutes
Calories: 386
Protein: 15 Grams
Fat: 11 Grams
Carbs: 59 Grams
Ingredients:

- 1 Sweet Onion, Sliced Thick
- 1 Eggplant, Sliced Thick
- 2 Zucchini, Sliced Lengthwise
- 2 Tablespoons Olive Oil
- 28 Ounces Canned tomatoes, Diced & Sodium Free
- 1 Cup Quartered, Canned & Water Packed Artichokes, Drained
- 2 Teaspoons Basil, Fresh & Chopped
- 2 Teaspoons Garlic, Minced
- 2 Teaspoons Oregano, Fresh & Chopped
- 12 Lasagna Noodles, Whole Grain & No Boil
- ¼ Teaspoon Red Pepper Flakes
- ¾ Cup Asiago Cheese, Grated

Directions:

1. Start by heating your oven to 400, and then get out a baking sheet. Line it with foil before placing it to the side.
2. Get out a large bowl and toss your zucchini, yellow squash, eggplant, onion and olive oil, making sure it's coated well.
3. Arrange your vegetables on the baking sheet, roasting for twenty minutes. They should be lightly caramelized and tender.
4. Chop your roasted vegetables before placing them in a bowl.
5. Stir in your garlic, basil, oregano, artichoke hearts, tomatoes and red pepper flakes, spooning a quarter of this mixture in the bottom of a nine by thirteen baking dish. Arrange four lasagna noodles over this sauce, and continue by alternating it. Sprinkle with asiago cheese on top, baking for a half hour.
6. Allow it to cool for fifteen minutes before slicing to serve.

Chili Calamari

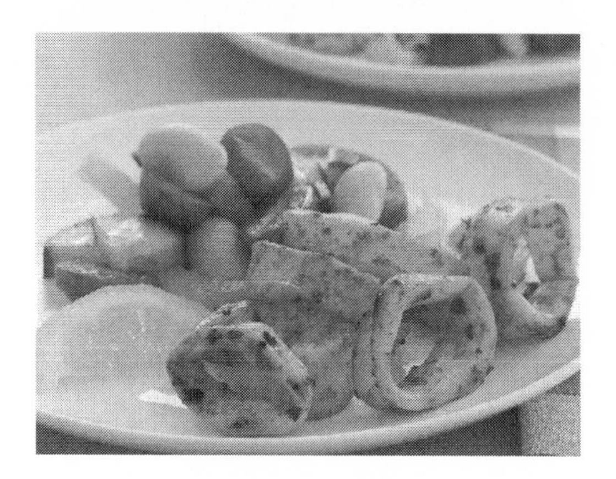

Serves: 4
Time: 1 Hour 20 Minutes
Calories: 222
Protein: 27 Grams
Fat: 10 Grams
Carbs: 6 Grams
Ingredients:

- 1 Lime, Juiced & Zested
- 2 Tablespoons Olive Oil
- 1 Teaspoon Chili Powder
- ½ Teaspoon Cumin, Ground
- ¼ Teaspoon Sea Salt, Fine
- ¼ Teaspoon Black Pepper
- 2 Tablespoons Cilantro, Fresh & Chopped
- 2 Tablespoons Red Bell Pepper, Minced
- 1 ½ lbs. Squid, Cleaned, Split Open & Cut into ½ Inch Rounds

Directions:

1. Get out a bowl and mix your chili powder, cumin, lime juice, lime zest, olive oil, salt and pepper together. Add in your squid, and make sure it's well coated. Cover and allow it to marinate in the fridge for an hour.
2. Preheat your oven to a broil, and get out a baking sheet. Lay your squid on your baking sheet, broiling for eight minutes. You'll need to turn once in this time, and it should be tender.
3. Garnish with red bell pepper and cilantro before serving.

Scallops in a Citrus Sauce

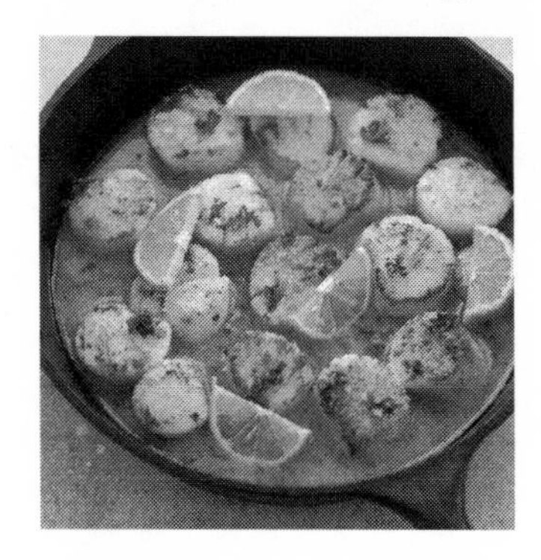

Serves: 4
Time: 25 Minutes
Calories: 207
Protein: 26 Grams
Fat: 4 Grams
Carbs: 17 Grams
Ingredients:

- 2 Teaspoons Olive Oil
- 1 Shallot, Minced
- 20 Sea Scallops, Cleaned
- 1 Teaspoon Lime Zest
- 1 Tablespoon Lemon Zest
- 2 Teaspoons Orange Zest
- 1 Tablespoon Basil, Fresh & Chopped
- ½ Cup Orange Juice, Fresh
- 2 Tablespoons Lemon Juice, Fresh
- 2 Tablespoons Honey, Raw
- 1 Tablespoon Greek Yogurt, Plain
- ½ Teaspoon Sea Salt, Fine

Directions:

1. Get out a large skillet and heat up your olive oil over medium-high heat. Add in your shallot, and sauté for a minute. They should soften.
2. Add your scallops in, searing for five minutes. Turn once during this time. They should be tender.
3. Push your scallops to the edge of the skillet, stirring in your three zests, basil, lemon juice and orange juice. Simmer for three minutes.
4. Whisk in your yogurt, honey and sea salt. Cook for four minutes. Coat your scallops in the sauce before serving warm.

Pork Chops & Wild Mushrooms

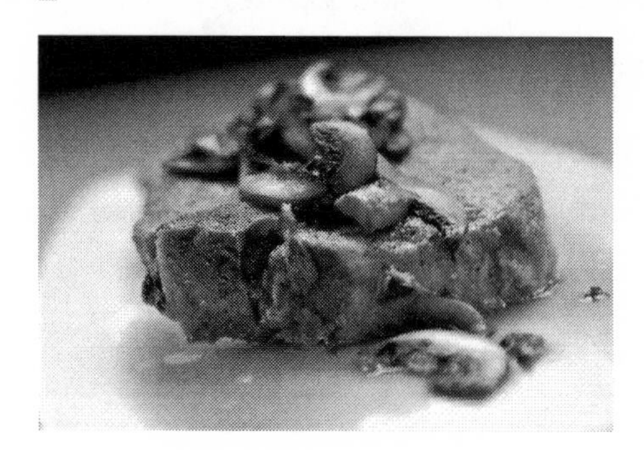

Serves: 4
Time: 35 Minutes
Calories: 308
Protein: 33 Grams
Fat: 17 Grams
Carbs: 7 Grams
Ingredients:

- 1 Tablespoon Olive Oil
- 4 Pork Chops, Center Cut, Bone In & 5 Ounces Each
- 1/4 Teaspoon Sea Salt, Fine
- 1/4 Teaspoon Black Pepper
- 1 Sweet Onion, Chopped
- 1 lb. Wild Mushrooms, Sliced
- 2 Teaspoons Garlic, Minced
- 1 Teaspoon Thyme, Fresh & Chopped
- 1/2 Cup Chicken Stock, Sodium Free

Directions:

1. Start by patting your pork chops dry using paper towel. Sprinkle your salt and pepper over them, and then get out a large skillet.

2. Place your skillet over medium-high heat and add in your olive oil. Once your oil is hot, add in your pork chops and cook for another six minutes. Brown them on both sides, and then put them on a plate.
3. Using the same skillet sauté your garlic and onion for three minutes. They should be fragrant and softened.
4. Add in your mushrooms and thyme, cooking for six more minutes. Your mushrooms should be tender and lightly caramelized.
5. Return your pork chops to the skillet and add in your chicken stock. Bring it to a boil while covered, and reduce your heat to low. Allow it to simmer for ten more minutes before serving warm.

Trout & Greens

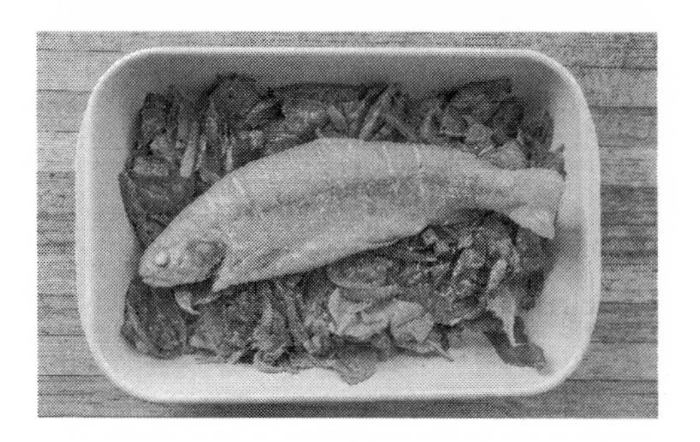

Serves: 4
Time: 20 Minutes
Calories: 315
Protein: 39 Grams
Fat: 14 Grams
Carbs: 6 Grams
Ingredients:

- 2 Teaspoons Olive Oil + More for Greasing
- 2 Cups Swiss Chard, Chopped
- 2 Cups Kale, Chopped
- ½ Sweet Onion, Sliced Thin
- 4 Trout Fillets, Skin On & 5 Ounces Each
- 1 Lemon, Zested
- ¼ Teaspoon Sea Salt, Fine
- ¼ Teaspoon Black Pepper

Directions:

1. Start by heating your oven to 375, and then grease a nine by thirteen inch baking dish using olive oil. Arrange your swiss chard, kale and onion on the bottom.

2. Top with greens and then place your fish on top. Make sure the skin side is up, and drizzle with lemon juice and olive oil. Season with salt and pepper before baking for fifteen minutes. Serve with lemon zest.

Tuscan Chicken with Rice

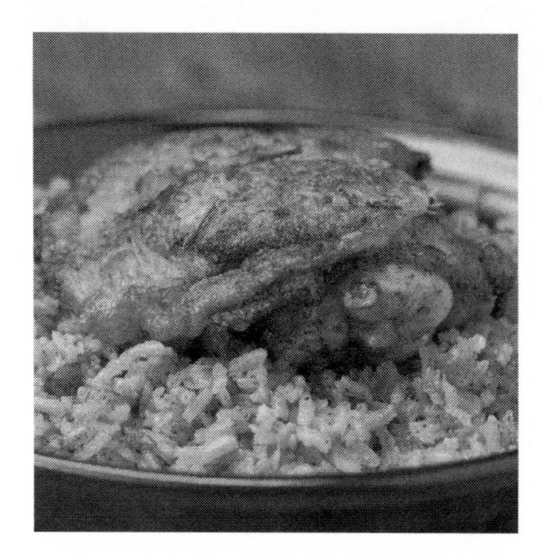

Serves: 6
Time: 1 Hour 5 Minutes
Calories; 320
Protein: 29 Grams
Fat: 11 Grams
Carbs: 29 Grams
Ingredients:

- ¾ Cup Brown Rice
- 1 Cup Cherry Tomatoes, Halved
- 1 Yellow Bell Pepper, Diced
- ½ Red Onion, Chopped
- ¼ Cup Kalamata Olives, Sliced
- 4 Chicken Breasts, 4 Ounces Each, Boneless, Skinless, & Cut into 3 Pieces
- 2 Teaspoons Oregano, Fresh & Chopped
- 1 Teaspoon Garlic Powder
- ½ Cup Goat Cheese, Crumbled
- 2 Cups Chicken Stock, Sodium Free
- ½ Lemon, Juiced
- 1 Tablespoon Parsley, Fresh & Chopped

Directions:

1. Start by heating your oven to 350, and then get out a bowl. Mix together your cherry tomatoes, red onion, bell pepper, olive sand brown rice. Spoon this mxi into a nine by thirteen inch baking dish.
2. Lay your chicken on top, and then season with garlic powder and oregano. Pour the lemon juice and chicken stock in.
3. Cover and bake for forty to forty-five minutes. The rice should be cooked as well as the chicken. Fluff before serving with goat cheese and parsley.

Pork Chops & Peaches

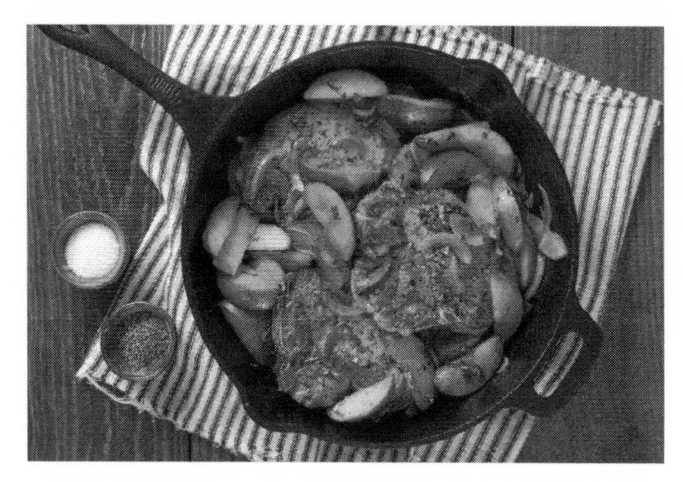

Serves: 4
Time: 45 Minutes
Calories; 307
Protein: 38 Grams
Fat: 12 Grams
Carbs: 10 Grams
Ingredients:

- ½ Fennel Bulb, Chopped in 1 Inch Chunks
- 4 Pork Chops, Boneless, 5 Ounces Each & Trimmed
- 2 Tablespoons Olive Oil, Divided + More for Greasing
- 2 Peaches, Pitted & Quartered
- 1 Sweet Onion, Peeled & Sliced Thin
- 2 Tablespoons Balsamic Vinegar
- 1 Teaspoon Thyme, Fresh & Chopped
- 1/4 Teaspoon Sea Salt, Fine
- ¼ Teaspoon Black Pepper

Directions:

1. Heat your oven to 400, and then get out a nine by thirteen inch baking dish. Make sure to grease it with olive oil before placing it to the side. Season your pork chops with salt and pepper.
2. Get out a bowl and toss your onion, peaches, fennel, thyme, balsamic vinegar, a tablespoon of olive oil and thyme. Roast them in your baking dish for twenty minutes.
3. Get out a skillet, placing it over medium-high heat, and heat up your remaining oil.
4. Add in your pork chops, searing for two minutes per side.
5. Take your vegetables out of the oven and stir them. Place the pork chops on top, and then roast for another ten minutes. Your pork should be cooked all the way through.

Side Dish Recipes

Artichoke Hearts

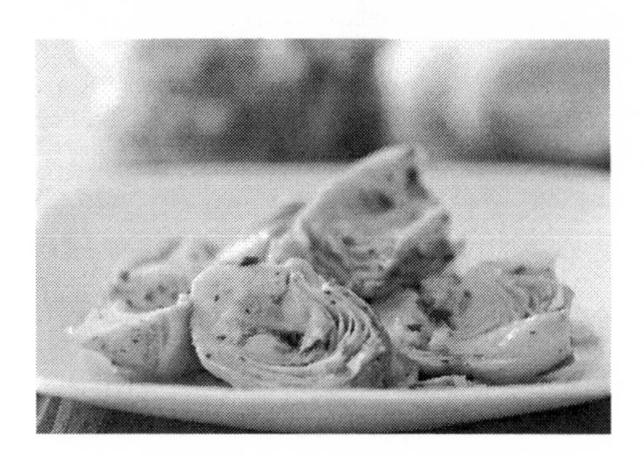

Serves: 4
Time: 30 Minute
Calories: 415
Protein: 12 Grams
Fat: 31 Grams
Carbs: 29 Grams
Ingredients:

- ¾ Cup Cornmeal
- 1/3 Cup Parmesan Cheese, Finely Grated
- 1 Teaspoon Garlic Powder
- 1 Teaspoon Sea Salt, Fine
- ½ Teaspoon Rosemary
- ½ Teaspoon Paprika
- ¼ Teaspoon Black Pepper
- 2 Eggs, Beaten Lightly
- ½ Cup Olive Oil, Divided
- 14 Ounces Artichoke Hearts, Canned & Drained

Directions:

1. Start by preheating your oven to 400, and then get out a wide but shallow bowl. In this bowl combine your garlic, slat, rosemary, parmesan, paprika and pepper. Make sure it's mixed well.
2. Mix your eggs and ¼ cup of olive oil together. Drain your artichoke hearts and add them to the egg mixture, stirring to combine.
3. Get out a rimmed baking sheet and oil it with the remaining olive oil.
4. Remove your artichoke hearts from the egg mixture, and roll them in the cornmeal mixture until they are evenly coated. Place them on your baking sheet, and then bake for fifteen twenty minutes. They should be lightly browned. Serve hot.

Roasted Baby Potatoes

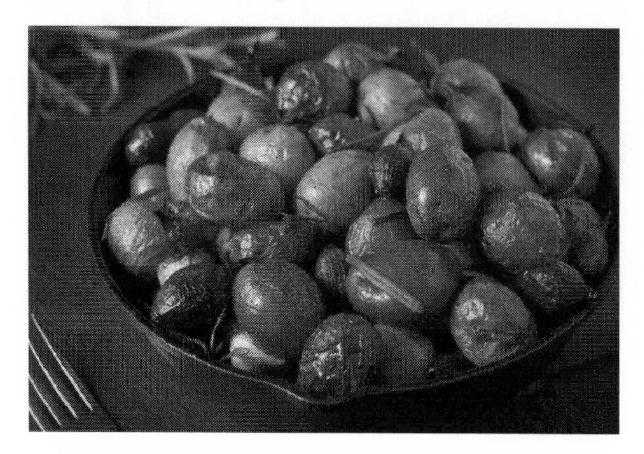

Serves: 4
Time: 45 Minutes
Calories: 225
Protein: 5 Grams
Fat: 7 Grams
Carbs: 37 Grams
Ingredients:

- 2 lbs. Red Potatoes, Scrubbed & Cut into Wedges
- 1 Teaspoon Sweet Paprika
- 1 Teaspoon Garlic Powder
- 2 Teaspoon Rosemary, Fresh & chopped
- 2 Tablespoons Olive Oil
- ½ Teaspoon Sea Salt, Fine
- ½ Teaspoon Black Pepper

Directions:

1. Start by heating your oven to 400, and then get out a baking sheet. Line your baking sheet with foil before setting it to the side.
2. Get out a large bowl and toss your olive oil, rosemary, potatoes, paprika, garlic powder, sea salt and pepper.

3. Spread your potatoes out on the baking sheet in a single layer, and bake for thirty-five minutes. They should be tender and golden brown. Serve warm.

Scalloped Tomatoes

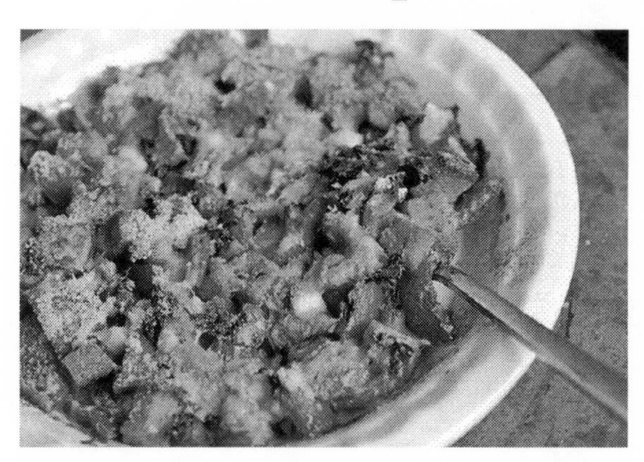

Serves: 4
Time: 55 Minutes
Calories: 127
Protein: 5 Grams
Fat: 6 Grams
Carbs: 16 Grams
Ingredients:

- 1 Olive Oil, Divided
- 2 Slices Whole Wheat, Cut into ½ Inch Cubes
- 2 ¼ lbs. Tomatoes, Cut into Eights
- 2 Tablespoons Asiago Cheese, Shredded
- ¼ Cup Basil, Fresh & Chopped
- 1 Tablespoon Garlic, Minced
- ¼ Teaspoon Sea Salt, Fine
- ¼ Teaspoon Black Pepper

Directions:

1. Start by heating the oven to 350, and then get out an eight by eight inch baking dish. Grease it with ½ teaspoon olive oil before setting the baking dish to the side.
2. Get out a large skillet, placing it over medium-high heat and heating up the remaining olive oil.
3. Add in your bread cubes and sauté for four minutes. They should be golden on all sides, and then add in your garlic. Stir and cook for two minutes. Add in your tomatoes and cook for another two minutes.
4. Remove it form the skillet, and the season with salt and pepper. Stir in your basil, and then transfer to your baking dish.
5. Sprinkle your asiago cheese on the top, and bake for a half hour.

Brussel Sprouts & Pistachios

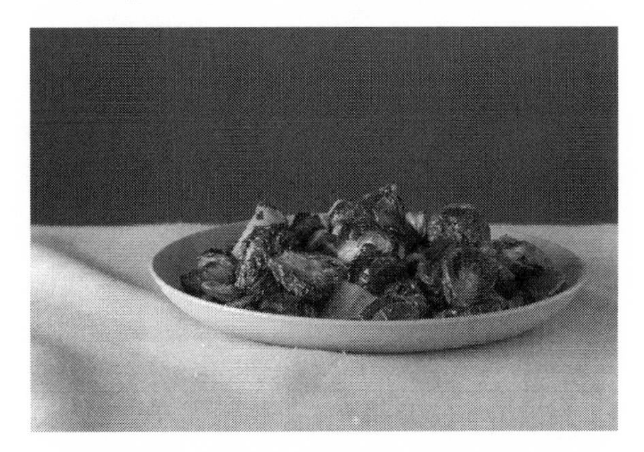

Serves: 4
Time: 30 Minutes
Calories: 126
Protein: 6 Grams
Fat: 7 Grams
Carbs: 14 Grams
Ingredients:

- 1 lb. Brussel Sprouts, Trimmed & Halved Lengthwise
- 4 Shallots, Peeled & Quartered
- ½ Cup Pistachios, Roasted & Chopped
- 1/2 Lemon, Zested & Juiced
- ¼ Teaspoon Sea Salt, Fine
- ¼ Teaspoon Black Pepper
- 1 Tablespoon Olive Oil

Directions:

1. Start by heating your oven to 400, and then get out a baking sheet. Line it with foil before placing it to the side.
2. Get out a bowl and toss your shallots and brussels sprouts in olive oil, making sure that it's well coated.

3. Season with salt and pepper before spreading your vegetables out on the pan.
4. Bake for fifteen minutes. Your vegetables should be lightly caramelized as well as tender.
5. Take it out of the oven and toss with lemon zest, lemon juice and pistachios before serving.

Mashed Celeriac

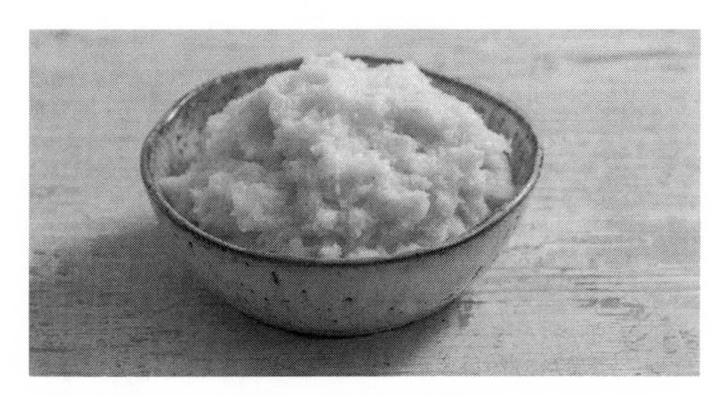

Serves: 4
Time: 30 Minutes
Calories: 136
Protein: 4 Grams
Fat: 3 Grams
Carbs: 26 Grams
Ingredients:

- 2 Celery Roots, Washed, Peeled & Diced
- 1 Tablespoon Honey, Raw
- 2 Teaspoons Olive Oil
- ½ Teaspoon Nutmeg, Ground
- ¼ Teaspoon Sea Salt, Fine
- ¼ Teaspoon Black Pepper

Directions:

1. Start by heating your oven to 400, and then get out a baking sheet. Line it with foil before setting it to the side.
2. Get out a bowl and mix your olive oil and celery root, spreading it out on the baking sheet. Roast for twenty minutes. It should be lightly caramelized and tender, and then place it back in the bowl.

3. Add your honey and nutmeg in before mashing with a potato masher. Season with salt and pepper before serving.

Fennel Wild Rice

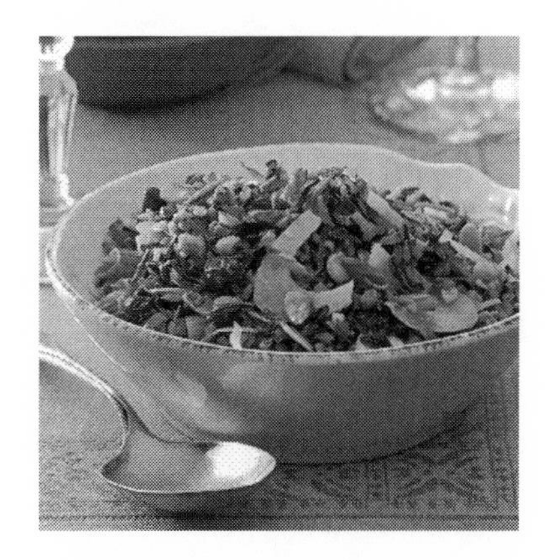

Serves: 6
Time: 25 Minutes
Calories: 222
Protein: 8 Grams
Fat: 3 Grams
Carbs: 43 Grams
Ingredients:

- 1 Tablespoon Parsley, Fresh & Chopped
- 2 Cups Wild Rice, Cooked
- 1 Cup Fennel, Diced
- 1 Tablespoon Olive Oil
- ½ Cup Sweet Onion, Chopped
- ½ Red Bell Pepper, Diced Fine
- ¼ Teaspoon Sea Salt, Fine
- ¼ Teaspoon Black Pepper

Directions:

1. Get out a skillet and place it over medium-high heat. Heat up your olive oil and add in your onion, red bell pepper and fennel. Sauté for six minutes. It should become tender.

2. Stir in your wild rice, and cook for five minutes, and then add in your parsley. Season with salt and pepper before serving warm.

Parmesan Broccoli

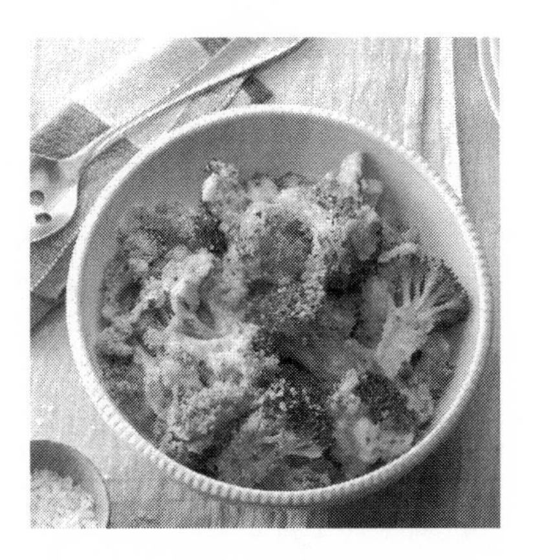

Serves: 4
Time: 20 Minutes
Calories: 154
Protein: 9 Grams
Fat: 11 Grams
Carbs: 10 Grams
Ingredients:

- 2 Teaspoons Garlic, Minced
- 2 Tablespoons Olive Oil + More for Greasing the Baking Sheet
- 2 Heads Broccoli, Cut into Florets
- 1 Lemon, Zested & Juiced
- ½ Cup Parmesan Cheese, Grated
- Sea Salt to Taste

Directions:

1. Start by heating your oven to 400, and then get out a baking sheet. Grease with olive oil before setting it to the side.
2. Get a large bowl out and toss your broccoli with garlic, lemon zest, lemon juice, olive oil and sea salt. Spread this mixture on the baking sheet. Make sure it's on a single layer, and then sprinkle with Parmesan cheese.

3. Bake for ten minutes. Your broccoli should be tender, and then serve warm.

Dessert Recipes

Cherry Clafoutis

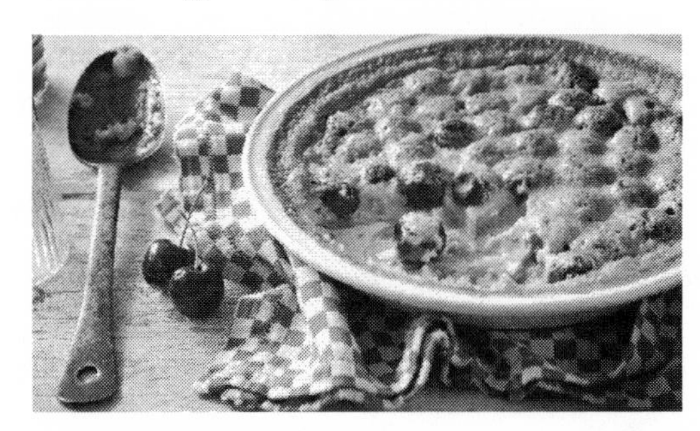

Serves: 4
Time: 45 Minutes
Calories: 407
Protein: 10 Grams
Fat: 16 Grams
Carbs: 57 Grams
Ingredients:

- 2 Tablespoons Butter, Room Temperature
- ½ Cup Almonds, Unsalted & Ground
- 1 ¼ Cups Milk
- 2 Eggs
- ½ Cup Sugar, Divided
- ½ Cup All Purpose Flour
- 1 Tablespoon Vanilla Extract, Pure
- 3 Cups cherries, Pitted
- 1/8 Teaspoon Sea Salt, Fine

Directions:

1. Start by heating your oven to 350, and then get out a nine inch pie pan. Brush it down with butter, sprinkling your ground almonds on the bottom.

2. Mix your milk, eggs, vanilla, ¼ cup of sugar, flour, and salt in a blender, pureeing until smooth.
3. Pour this batter into your pie plate, and arrange your cherries over the batter. Sprinkle your remaining sugar on top, and bake for thirty-five to forty-five minutes. It should be golden brown.
4. Allow it to cool for at least ten minutes before serving.

Stuffed Figs

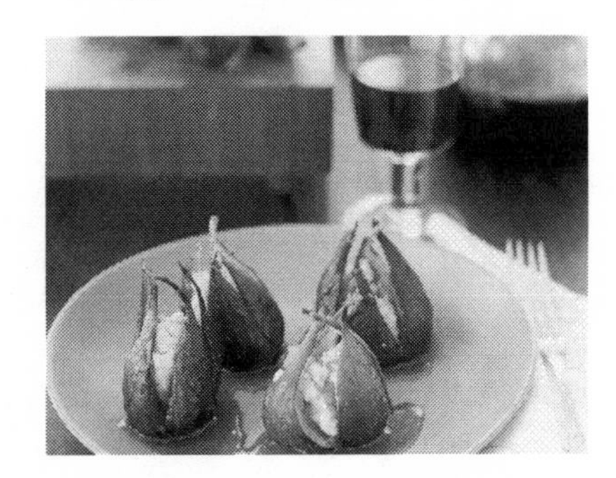

Serves: 6
Time: 20 Minutes
Calories: 209
Protein: 8 Grams
Fat: 9 Grams
Carbs: 27 Grams
Ingredients:

- 20 Almonds, Chopped
- 2 Tablespoons Honey, Raw
- 4 Ounces Goat Cheese, Divided
- 10 Fresh Figs, Halved

Directions:

1. Start by preheating your oven's broiler to high.
2. Get out a baking sheet and place your figs with the cut side up. Sprinkle each with ½ teaspoon of goat cheese and a teaspoon of almond. Broil for two to three minutes, and then allow them to cool for five minutes before drizzling with honey to serve.

Honey Panna Cotta

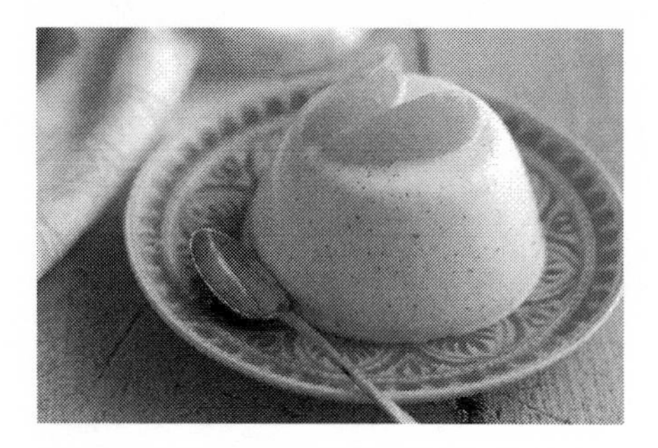

Serves: 6 **Time:** 4 Hours 15 Minutes
Calories: 274
Protein: 1 Gram
Fat: 22 Grams
Carbs: 19 Grams
Ingredients:

- 4 Teaspoons Gelatin, Unflavored
- 3 Cups Heavy Whipping Cream
- ½ Teaspoon Almond Extract
- 6 Tablespoons Honey, Raw
- 1 Teaspoon Vanilla Extract, Pure

Directions:

1. Get out a bowl and stir your gelatin with a half a cup of heavy cream, setting it to the side.
2. Get out a saucepan, placing it over medium-high heat and heating up your remaining cream. It should be just below boiling. Remove it from heat, and then whisk in your almond extract, honey and vanilla extract. You should whisk for three minutes until the honey fully dissolves.
3. Whisk in the gelatin mixture, and then pour into a four coup serving dish.
4. Place it in the fridge for at least four hours to set.

5. Loosen the panna cotta bay running a knife around the edge and turn it over to get the pudding out to serve chilled.

Strawberry Chia Pudding

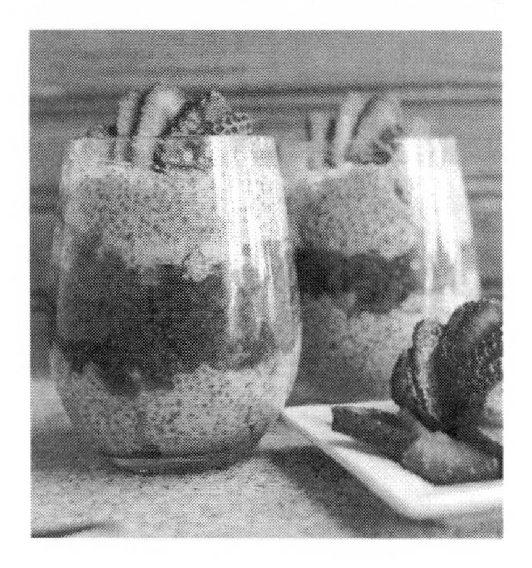

Serves: 4
Time: 4 Hours 5 Minutes
Calories: 108
Protein: 3 Grams
Fat: 4 Grams
Carbs: 18 Grams
Ingredients:

- ¼ Cup Chia Seeds
- 2 Cups Almond Milk, Unsweetened
- 2 Cups Strawberries, Fresh & Sliced
- 1 Tablespoon Vanilla Extract, Pure
- 2 Tablespoons Honey, Raw

Directions:

1. Get out a bowl and mix your vanilla, honey, almond milk and chia seeds.
2. Refrigerate for four hours, and then serve topped with strawberries.

Gingered Melon

Serves: 4
Time: 15 Minutes
Calories: 91
Protein: 1 Gram
Fat: 0 Grams
Carbs: 24 Grams
Ingredients:

- 2 Cups Watermelon Chunks, 1 Inch
- ½ Cantaloupe, Peeled & Chopped into 1 Inch Chunks
- 2 Tablespoons Honey, Raw
- 2 Cups Honeydew Melon Chunks, 1 Inch
- 2 Inch Piece of Ginger, Peeled, Grated & Juice Reserved

Directions:

1. Get out a bowl and mix your honeydew, watermelon and cantaloupe.
2. Add in your ginger juice and honey before serving chilled.

Spiced Pear with Applesauce

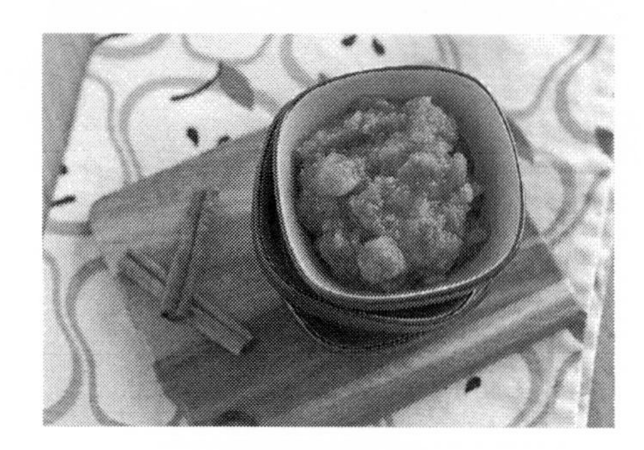

Serves: 4
Time: 15 Minutes
Calories: 202
Protein: 1 Gram
Fat: 1 Gram
Carbs: 53 Grams
Ingredients:

- ¼ Teaspoon Nutmeg, Ground
- ½ Teaspoon Cinnamon, Ground
- 2 Tablespoons Honey, Raw
- ¼ Cup Water
- 2 Tart Apples, Peeled, Cored & Chopped
- 1/8 Teaspoon Cloves, Ground
- 4 Pears, Peeled, Cored & Chopped
- ¼ Cup Water

Directions:

1. Place a saucepan over medium heat, adding in your ingredients. Cover the pan and bring it to a boil. Reduce the heat to low, cooking for twenty minutes. The fruit should soften.
2. Remove it form the pot, and then mash until mostly smooth.
3. Chill before serving.

Conclusion

Now you know everything you need to understand and get started with the Mediterranean diet! There's nothing to stop you from your weight loss and health goals on this diet. Just follow the simple tips and tricks provided to you, and start with a few recipes that sound great. They're sure to become family favorites in no time at all! Any dietary change can be hard at first, but with delicious, new recipes, every day becomes a little easier.